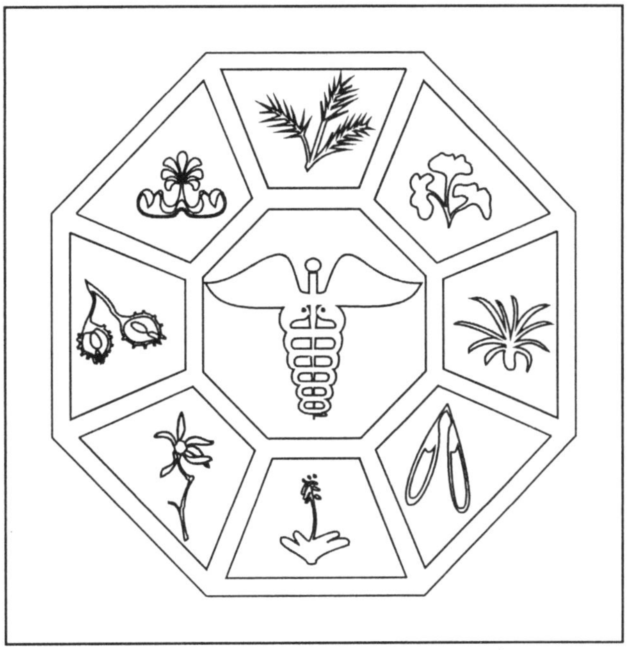

Tijuana Clinics Alternative Therapies

A 23 Year Analysis

By Sally Wolper

Tijuana Clinics
by Sally Wolper

PUBLISHED BY:
Promotion Publishing
3368-F Governor Dr. #144
San Diego, CA 92122

1-800-231-1776

ISBN 1-887314-03-2

Photography by
Steve Lopushinsky
Turville Photography
Orange, California

Desktop Publishing by
Suzanne Merritt
Carlsbad, California

Notice:

Mexican laws may change periodically regarding the various medicines used in the Alternative Therapy Clinics. Neither the author nor the publisher shall take any responsibility for any change that may take place.

A Tribute to Mexico

From a town that seems
out of the past come
probably the most
advanced and
sophisticated treatments
for cancer.

Some of the greatest
physicians in the world are
now gathered together in
one place,
Tijuana, Mexico.

Mexico has welcomed
these clinicians with open
hearts and open minds.

Thank you, Mexico, for
being a good neighbor.

This book is dedicated to Gil Greer and Grandma.

Acknowledgments

My sincere thanks and appreciation to the International Association of Cancer Victors and Friends of Santa Barbara, California. This book is mostly what the late Los Angeles Chapter's President, Betty Lee Morales, once taught me, and what the IACVF is all about: "A better way to treat cancer."

Many thanks to all the Tijuana Clinics' cancer patients who out lived their home town doctors' prognosises, convincing me that the cure for cancer may lie in strange and unfamiliar therapies.

And to John Perkins and Christopher Hartman of Promotion Publishing who had the courage, integrity and willingness to publish and promote, making available to public, this type of informed choice book.

Introduction

The word "cancer" is alarming and even more alarming is that one out of every three people in the United States will get cancer. The symptom of cancer is usually a tumor which is an advance sign of the disease. The tumor is usually diagnosed clinically by palpation, X-ray and/or biopsy. After aggressive treatment—surgery, radiation, chemotherapy and hormones—prognosis is still grim. No wonder people are looking seriously at non-aggressive, host-saving alternatives.

Some of these alternatives lie across the Mexican border in Tijuana, Mexico. The physicians in the Tijuana Clinics have one main thing in common: to treat cancer and other diseases with "non-toxic" and "non-aggressive" therapies. For most who choose these treatments, they are not just desperate people looking for a last attempt. They really believe this is a better way to treat cancer.

Author's Note:

Many people come to the alternative clinics in Tijuana, Mexico for treatment because of the wide variety of international therapies available there.

The clinics may or may not have specific procedures, maintain specific standards and/or keep statistics according to the United States ICD-9 medical standards.

Therefore, neither the author nor the publisher make any recommendations nor assume any responsibility in regard to treatment in Mexico.

This book is written as an informative publication and is not intended to be used in lieu of doctor's treatment.

If you are ill, please contact your physician and your metabolic physician.

Table of Contents

Foreword

When you think of the word "pioneer" you might think of someone who did it first. When I think of metabolic physicians and nutritionists I think they have been pioneers for hundreds of years. It is time these pioneers came of age. Perhaps it would help if we called them scientific nutritional chemists.

When you think of a nutritionist you might imagine a white-coated person preparing a hospital's weekly menu. The whole idea of a nutritionist coming to the forefront of medicine and curing cancer with a diet has been almost inconceivable until now.

How could it be that a nutritionist could know more about cancer than a doctor?

Through no fault of his own the average doctor has rarely been made aware of the importance of the chemical compositions that we put into our bodies—that stuff we call food. It has almost been taken for granted that this incredible body could and would somehow take care of itself. Some homeostasis would make everything okay.

After years of abusing our bodies with wrong foods, the body finally gives up and it is never "just okay" again.

Our freedom to choose whatever foods suit our fancy and put unthought-about food concoctions into our bodies could just be setting us up as candidates for disease. We don't even follow the supposed well-balanced diet with any consistency.

It is difficult to understand how and why we have been allowed to follow the wrong human food formulas for so long and even make up our own formulas. Food formulas should be a priority for our existence. Someone should make it a science.

What else have nutritionists and metabolic physicians discovered that has given them the right to take the position of cancer doctor?

Somehow nutritionists, metabolic physicians, chiropractors, colon therapists and herbalists all seem to have studied that fasting and cleansing the colon can help to repair the body.

They have also discovered that if normal blood profiles are obtained from people in a population that gets sick, then these normals need to be re-evaluated. Average doesn't necessarily mean normal.

Another plus for the patients and doctors of nutritional therapy is that there are no secrets kept from the patients about their health. Patients often carry around with them copies of their own medical records. Because the metabolic patient's getting well depends upon his own understanding and at-home follow-up care, the nutritional physician spends much time defining, explaining, and teaching this new approach to his patients. This honesty and intimacy has created a new kind of bond between doctor and patient.

Author's Story

Sally Wolper, H.R.T.
(Health Record
Technician) and student of
A.R.T. (Accredited Record
Technician).

I have been no stranger to cancer. My adopted father died of this terrible disease when I was 17. His death and other circumstances led me into a foster home. Although very wealthy, my foster father could not stop the cancer that my foster mother was to get a few years later.

At 20, I worked at AVON Products in Pasadena as an artist. I married and later divorced. With little clerical experience, I gained employment with a medical group working the graveyard shift in the emergency room. I found that I enjoyed the medical world and have worked in that area ever since.

It was while employed at an industrial clinic in 1964 that a doctor befriended me. I respected this man because of his open-mindedness and dislike for the prejudices of the world. In 1972 he became ill with cancer at the age of 48. Refusing the regular orthodox treatments, he remained at home. During this same time, some of my other friends became ill with the symptoms of cancer.

My brother had given me a paperback book called *Does Dr. Max Gerson Have A Cure For Cancer?* I was able to trace the book to the Cancer control Society on Berendo Street in Los Angeles.

Thinking that I could be of help to my friends, I bought several books about alternative cancer therapies and took them to my doctor friend. I was sure that he could interpret what was written in them, but it was difficult for him with his illness to read and comprehend these concepts. Unfortunately, I was unable to help any of my friends. Four of them died within a two year period. Another friend, that I did not know had cancer, was taking Kribiozen and getting over her cancer. Kribiozen is an alternative cancer therapy.

Watching my friends' illnesses and their deaths, I learned that a person's dignity must be maintained in life, sickness, and in death, and that these alternative therapies offered at least that. Because one friend did live after taking Kribiozen, I thought these therapies also offered some hope for a cure. It seemed worth looking into and I became interested in cancer and its cures.

I began to volunteer to work in the Cancer Control Society's booth at conventions and sometimes in the office, cutting out newspaper articles. Clipping out articles did not seem a very important job, but these articles collectively became a most valued library for future reference. Little did I know that I would someday refer back to some of those articles to write books.

My intentions were to only volunteer a few times, but here it is 23 years later. As the years went by I started transcribing convention speeches for the Cancer Control Journals and sometimes proof-reading speeches for the Cancer Control Journals and sometimes proof reading the journals before publication. Biographies of the speakers were made for the conventions and somehow I adopted that job. By this time I was a paid volunteer.

Also, in 1984, I started a Statistical Registry at the Cancer control Society. This registry is very much like the Tumor Registry, but it also includes other diseases. Using the ICD-9-CM (International Classification of diseases, 9th edition, Clinical Modification), a Disease Index Coding System was set up. This is the same one used by Tumor Registries and the minimal requirement of the JCAH (the Joint Commission for the Accreditation of Hospitals).

Of course the Cancer Control Society was not a hospital and did not have a Physicians' Index nor an Operations Index. However a Patients' Index was available for the convenience of having them in alphabetical order. The names have been given numbered folders for confidentiality. This Disease Index is enabling us to see which of the metabolic therapies are working best for different kinds of cancer and to see how many people have gotten over their cancer without using "orthodox" treatments. It also shows which kinds of therapies are best for other diseases as well.

For six years prior to 1984, I had worked as a Health Record Technician and a Medical Records Analysis Clerk for Metropolitan State Hospital in Norwalk, California. My job there consisted of reviewing discharged charts for deficiencies and coding the final diagnosis using the ICD-9-CM, putting the diagnosis on disease Index Cards and on computer. I was also responsible for the review of charts for special investigation. While employed at Metropolitan State Hospital, I received five Merit Awards from the State of California for implementing new and time-saving procedures in the Medical Record Department.

From 1984 to 1988 I worked for the State of California Youth Authority and presently, in 1995, work for the State of California Department of Rehabilitation.

In 1984 I had to have help with the biographies because I had a new job, drafting some 100 questions for the nurses to answer for their CEU (Continuing Education Units). These units are obtained by R.N.'s and L.V.N.'s by attending the Cancer Control Society's Annual Convention, the Doctors' Meeting, and by going on the Tijuana Clinics Tour.

AUTHOR'S COMMENT

I sincerely believe that there will come a time that all of these therapies that are used at the Tijuana clinics will be incorporated so that: American Biologics' high megavitamins and 24-hour intensive care will be available to anyone. Gerson's beautiful detoxification program and use of ozone, Hoxsey's advanced testing and their herbs will be utilized. Contreras's cleansing I.V. drip and spiritual and emotional healing will be a major part of treatment. Genesis West's growth hormone therapy will be considered for those who need it. Hospital Santa Monica's balancing I.V. drip and hydrogen peroxide will be a part of treatment. Manner's cocktail (I.V. drip) for building the body and attacking the tumor. Bio-electric medicine will be a consideration for anyone. Castillo's chelation and Bio-medical medicine's, homeopathics will be used, alternative dentistry will be part of medical therapy. Bio-Revives hyperthermia will become a part of therapy. I believe these treatments will become one treatment that will put the body into a suspended state of balance long enough until its own immune system, out of stress, can function at the highest possible level and the body will heal itself.

PART I

"If the doctors of today do not become the dietitians of tomorrow, the dietitians of today will become the doctors of tomorrow."
—Rockefeller Institute of Medical Research

Historic Clinics

How many clinics are there? Maybe one or two. Well, let's see—there's that Laetrile doctor and there's that herbal place."

Forty years ago there were only two, but well known, Tijuana Clinics. They had been there for a long time and may have suffered more fame and ridicule than all the other clinics put together, but permission and time were in their favor, and patient testimonials.

Metabolic therapy most famous for Laetrile

(1950's) Hospital Ernesto Contreras became famous under the direction of Dr. Ernesto Contreras after he treated a patient, Cecile Hoffman. She had come to him to ask if he would inject a substance that she had gotten from Canada for her cancer. You guessed it: Laetrile. After seeing the benefits of Laetrile, Dr. Contreras began using it on other patients. One of his most famous patients was Chad Green.

Clinic most famous for Hoxsey Herbal Tonic

(1950's) Bio-Medical, another clinic, moved to Tijuana from Texas, now under the direction of Mildred Nelson, R.N. She inherited the secret of the famous herbal Hoxsey tonic from John Hoxsey's grandson, Harry.

Dr. Ivy was best known for his Kribiozen.

(1960's) Sometime a little later, a Dr. Andrew Ivy was also having some success in Chicago treating cancer with a formula derived from a horse serum called Kribiozen.

Most famous for use of Laetrile and recently Venus Fly Trap.

(1970's) Dr. Hans Knieper of Hanover, Germany, started treating and/or counseling some well known personalities from America—Alisha Buttons, Fred MacMurray, Yul Brenner and most recently our President, Ronald Reagan. Dr. Nieper uses many modalities.

Most famous for experiments with Laetrile, enzymes and vitamin A and for using, in treatment, of what he calls "The Manner Cocktail," which consists of vitamins, DMSO and Laetrile in an I.V. drip.

(1970's) Another doctor from Chicago, with his students, was doing animal experiments using Laetrile, enzymes and vitamin A. Dr. Harold Manner, then head of the Bio-chemistry Department at Loyola University, with much opposition, still was successful in proving the benefits of Laetrile, enzymes and vitamin A on cancerous mice. But because there is a difference between men and mice, he wanted the opportunity to prove their effectiveness on human beings. The Manner Clinic in Tijuana is one of 200 clinics around the world that had at one time used the Manner Therapy.

Most famous for its carrot juice, coffee enemas and recently ozone.

(1970's) About the same time, a lady by the name of Jackie Davison had written a book, *Cancer Winner,* about how she had cured herself of melanoma cancer by following the instructions in a book by Dr. Max Gerson called *The Gerson Therapy—50 Case Histories*. Realizing the need to reinstate and continue the Gerson Therapy under clinical supervision, Charlotte Gerson Strauss, Dr. Gerson's daughter, opened a clinic in Las Playas, Mexico, the Gerson Institute.

Santa Maria was most famous for using megadoses of vitamins.

(1970's) A dentist, Dr. William Kelly, had treated and controlled his own cancer with diet and wrote a book called *One Answer to Cancer.* Another clinic emerged in Mexico using some of Dr. Kelley's protocols. The clinic was called "Santa Maria" and was soon to become famous when actor Steve McQueen made public the benefits he received there.

(1970's) Santa Maria was located 50 miles south of Tijuana. Some of the doctors from the clinic joined some other doctors from around the world and re-established in La Mesa, Mexico, near Tijuana.

American Biologics is most famous for integrating international protocols.

American Biologics (Dr. Robert Bradford) was responsible for integrating many modalities for the clinic. This clinic was the first to be built in Tijuana for the specific purpose of treating patients with metabolic therapy.

Most famous for cellular therapy

(1970's) Along came a clinic that saw a specific need for cellular therapy and Genesis West was created. They did not concentrate so much on cancer patients, but emphasized rejuvenation of the whole body for anyone desiring to improve their health and well being. They are now located in Las Playas, Mexico, near Tijuana. This clinic was first established by Andrew McNaughton.

Most famous for mind/body healing techniques: Bio-electric and Rife Frequency Machines.

(1980's) Soon the reputation of another doctor by the name of Gary Richer became evident as more and more patients began to report, "He's got something going." That something incorporated many modalities including Dr. Bernard Jensen's tissue cleansing program. He also included techniques and exercises that could allow patients to experience the power and control they have over their own minds and bodies. The use of Rife Sound Frequency has been the most recent intervention. The name of this clinic is American Metabolics.

Best known for use of biological modifiers.

(1980's) Dr. Yolanda Fraire, after working with the Bio-Medical (Hoxsey) Clinic for several years, wanted to become independent and opened her clinic in 1984. She began to use "biological modifiers"—non-toxic agents that she says are from the National Cancer Institutes fourth Other Treatment for Cancer list. In the 1990's she joined the Castillo Clinic as a homeopathic physician.

Clinic most famous for amino acid formulas.

Then came a man who seemed to be carrying a football and getting tackled all the time. His name was Jimmy Keller, and St. Jude's Clinic was opened in 1984. Amino acid formulas, along with cellular therapy, kinesiology and radionics played important roles in this clinic's treatment program.

Most famous for Donsbach University and Nutritional College, publication of self-help books, his specially formulated I.V. drips and use of hydrogen peroxide in treatment.

(1986) Another man's vision was to inform all people of their right to be self-educated regarding their own health. Dr. Kurt W. Donsbach did this by selling millions of self-help publications. He later opened a nutritional college in Huntington Beach and in 1986 he built Hospital Santa Monica, Rosarito Beach, Mexico.

PART II

Don't commit intellectual suicide by closing yourself off to alternative possibilities, for after all, if what you know and do now is killing you, then you are suffering from a lack of knowledge and wisdom, and the saving answer to your problem may be found in new and unfamiliar territories."
—Dr. Bernard Jensen

Tijuana Clinics

What is a Tijuana Clinic?

The Alternative Therapies Clinics in Tijuana, Mexico offer a wide range of international, non-toxic, and non-aggressive alternatives for the treatment of all diseases, not exclusively cancer.

When you come to Tijuana for the first time, just like in America, you will see many medical offices and buildings, many "clinicas". They may or may not be *alternative cancer clinics.*

What is mentioned in this book are the alternative therapies clinics. What makes them stand out from other clinics is that they are very diverse, using international medicines, medically considered to be non-toxic and non-aggressive. They are called *alternative* because patients, particularly the cancer patient, have the privilege to choose from all the therapies that are available, and do not have to use a toxic medicine.

In Baja, Mexico, the Homeopath, the Herbalist, the Natureopath and, the Allopath, all hold equal status.

They are allowed to treat and cure any disease. There is no one profession that has the right to claim a monopoly on someone's health.

Most of the people who come to Mexico for cancer and other therapies have a choice in types of physicians, products and the methodology of administration.

Advanced Center of Integrated Medicine (European Therapies)

Institute Allen W. Lloyd Building,
Ave. Pasio Tijuana #406-201, 2nd floor
at international border
Tijuana, Mexico 22320
For mailing: Advanced Center of Integrated Medicine
P.O. Box 926 Bonita, CA 91908
(800) 337-1917, Fax: 011-52-66-824920
011-52-66-804902, 011-52-66-828313

Dr. J. Jeffrey Freeman, M.D., A.A.F.P., is the founder of Advanced Center of Integrated Medicine.

The institute provides natural biological medical services. These services include non-toxic, non-invasive testing and treatments for degenerative diseases such as cancer, heart disease, neurological and spinal injuries, chronic fatigue syndrome, and also help for alcohol and drug addiction. Testing at the institute includes regular laboratory testing and additional tests like the Darkfield, Doppler and Phethysograph tests.

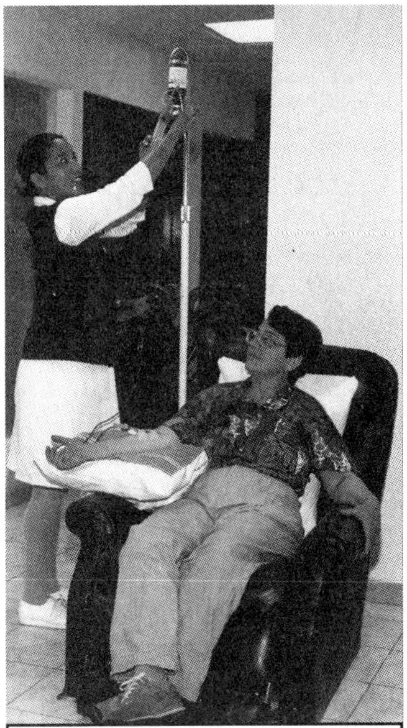

Blood Oxygenation

Natural biological therapies include detoxification, hyperthermia, bio-oxidative therapy, chelation therapy, major and minor autohemotherapy, I.V., I.M., hydrogen peroxide I.V. drips, and colon therapy.

A unique surgical procedure of spinal cord implants is performed in surgical quarters adjacent to the clinic. Dr. Freeman learned of these special procedures while studying in Mexico City.

Dr. Freeman has also developed a specialized program to fight heart disease and improve circulation to promote healing of other diseases. This program is called the "3-C's vascular cleanse". This cleanse helps remove plaque, and assists in the repair and strengthen vessels. The clinic also has set up a special clinic for prostate patients that has been "showing a very good success rate."

The medical staff at Advanced Center of Integrated Medicine have been trained in all aspects of European bio-oxidative therapies (ozone and hydrogen peroxide).

At the clinic, oxygen therapy methods are used, such as rectal insufflation and/or ozonated colonics according to the indication of the individual patient. They are used as anti bacterial, anti fungal and anti viral regulators.

Autohemotherapy (autophoresis) helps bind auto-immune antibodies. This is done by drawing approximately 50 cc of blood and passing it through an ultraviolet light and re-infusing it back into the patient. Autohemotherapy (autophoresis) helps bind auto-immune antibodies.

The institute believes that "establishing homeostasis is the key to wellness."

Advanced Center of Integrated Medicine is an out-patient clinic located near the American/Tijuana border. The base cost of therapy at Advanced Center of Integrated Medicine is approximately $3,800 a week.

Accommodations can be provided for in Rosarito Beach for $650 a month. Maid service is included.

- Specialty: prostate conditions, evaluation for spinal cord repair, alcohol and drug detoxification

Dr. Freeman, M.D.

Dr. Freeman, M.D., A. A. F. P., received his Medical Degree from the Autonome University of Guadalajara in 1972. He is a member of the American Academy of Family Physicians and the North American Hyperthermia Group.

He completed a residency at Baylor School of Medicine in Texas. He was at one time the Director of Medicine for the Department of Corrections in the State of Georgia and Osawattomie State Hospital, Kansas. Dr. Freeman is the Medical Director of the Advanced Center of Integrated Medicine in Tijuana, Mexico.

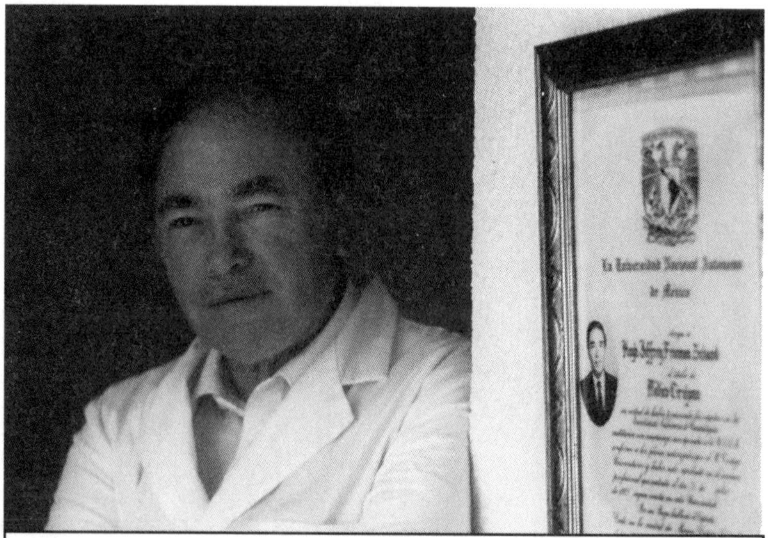

Dr. Jeffrey Freeman

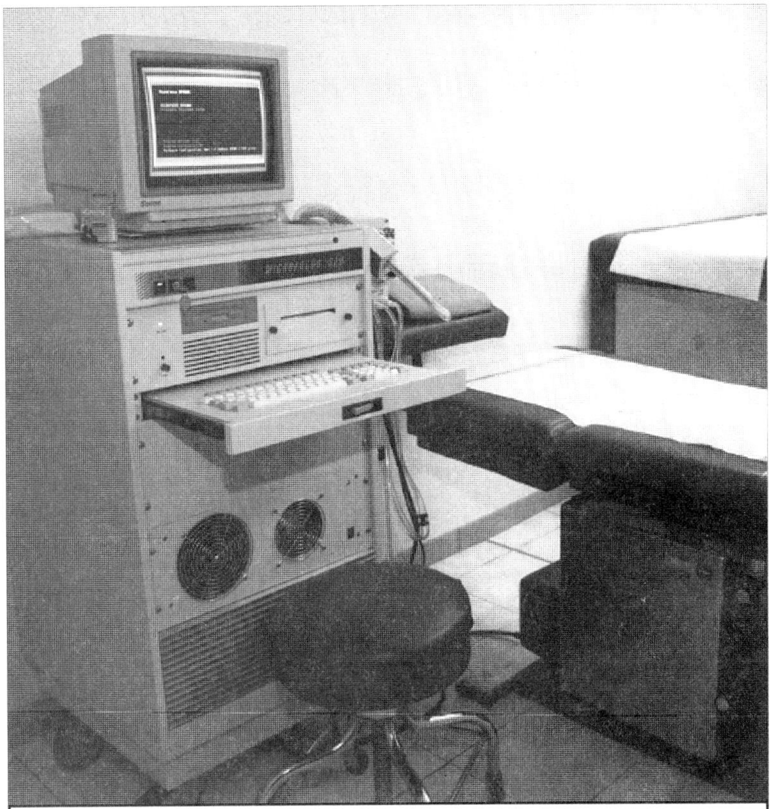

Enlarged Prostate Reduction Therapy Equipment

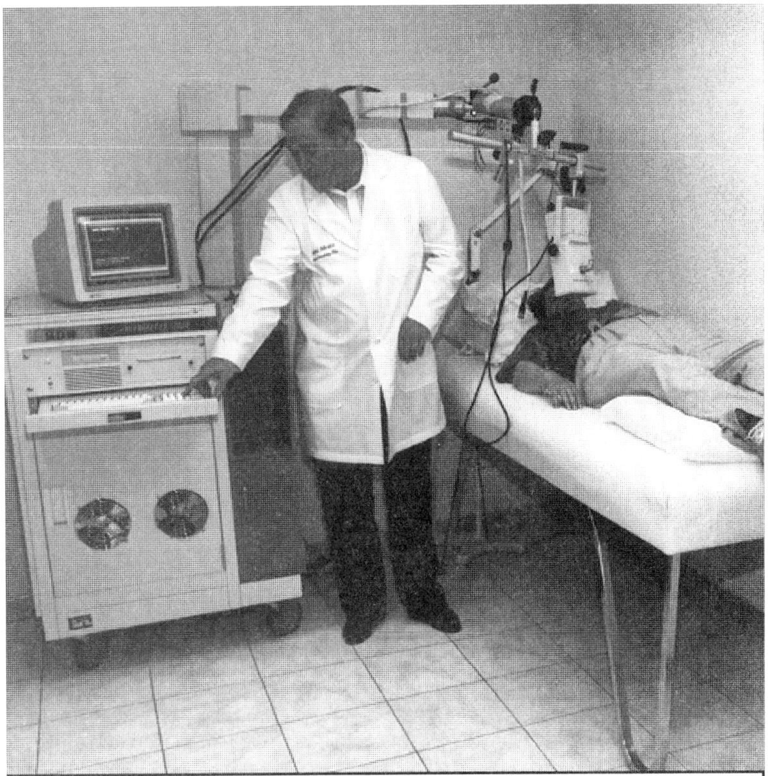

Hyperthermia Therapy

American Biologics

American Biologics (Integrated Metabolic Therapy)
Azucena #15 La Mesa, T.J. B.C., Mexico
For mailing: AB-Mexico 1180 Walnut Avenue
Chula Vista, CA 91911
(800) 227-4458
Inside California: (619) 429-8200
011-52-66-813171
FAX 011-52-66-816435

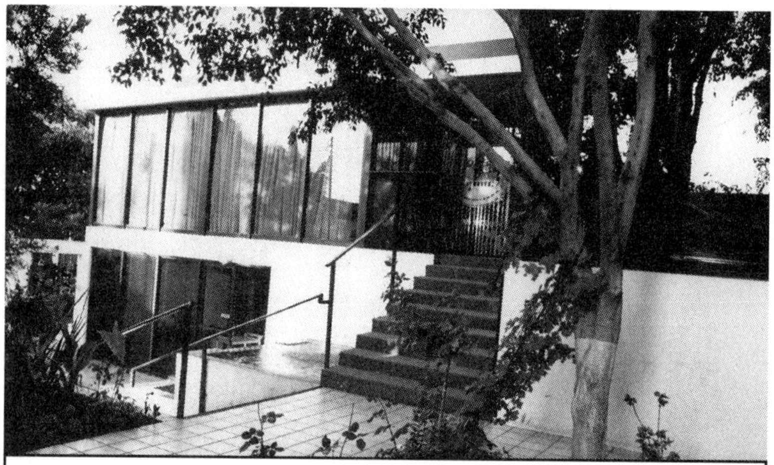

American Biologics' Hospital Entrance

The American Biologics-Mexico SA Research Hospital and Medical Center is a fully accredited and licensed general hospital/teaching facility with licensure for human research. As an accredited international hospital, staff privileges may be extended to physicians throughout the world upon request. Application information may be obtained by writing or calling American Biologics International headquarters at 1180 Walnut Avenue, Chula Vista, California 91911.

American Biologics has brought together many of the known alternative cancer therapies in one facility.

Dr. Bob Bradford, the facility's administrator and President of the Bradford Research Institute, could see the need and convenience of merging these therapies in one place. He has sought out what he believes is the best of what's working, the most often from around the world. He calls this implementing the treatment protocols for Individualized Integrated Metabolic Programs (IIMP).

Some of the therapies used at American Biologics are: Neihans cellular (growth-hormone) therapy; butyrate and staphage lysate for lymph system connected cancer; Bioelectric Medicine; aqueous solution injectable Laetrile; herbal poultices for non-surgical tumor removal; amino acid therapies; enzyme treatments; DMSO; gerovital (GH3); autogenous vaccines; Rodaquin; individualized nutritional and metabolic therapy; pH balancing; skeletal manipulation; EDTA (ethylene diamne tetra-acetic acid); chelation therapy (I.V. drip and oral); chondroiton sulfates; human interferon; colonic therapy; and detoxification. Also available are the standard or "orthodox" therapies and treatments which are integrated when jointly agreed upon by the medical staff and patients.

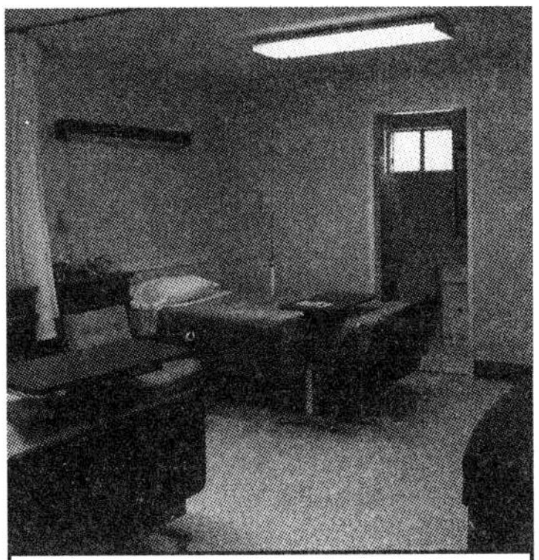

Patient's Room

Tests at American Biologics include the SMA 24 and Computerized Clinical Chemistry Correlation; the CAT scan; the M.I.T. (Metabolic Intolerance Test) for detecting food sensitivities; enzyme panels and amino acid profiles; computerized hair analysis for detection of nutritional mineral imbalances and heavy metal toxicity; and HLB Blood Test for daily monitoring of the effects of reactive oxygen toxic species (ROTS) on the blood. Standard blood assays for cancer including CEA and HCG are also available.

American Biologics Hospital and Medical Center is located three miles from the Tijuana border. Arrangements for clinical appointments and/or hospital reservation can be obtained by contacting AB-Mexico's international

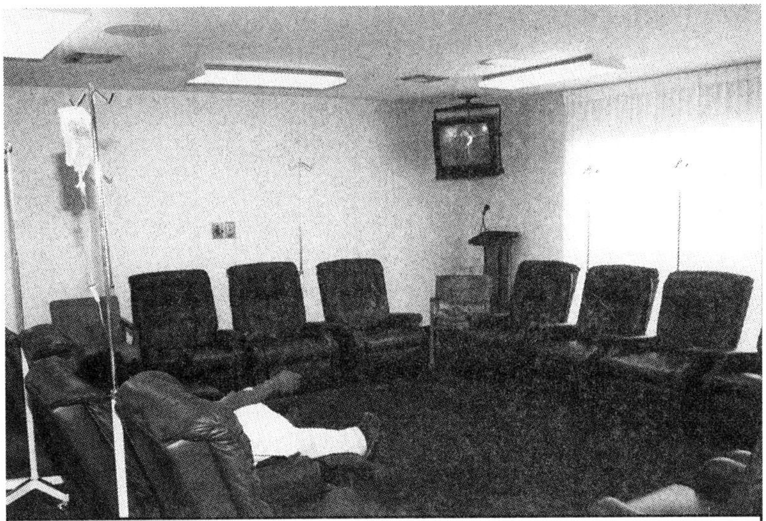

Chelation and Nutritional I.V. Room

headquarters, located in nearby Chula Vista, California. The approximate cost for a three week in-patient stay at American Biologics is approximately $13,000, and for an out-patient stay, $11,000.

- Specialty: brain, breast, cerebral palsy, multiple sclerosis, neurological disorders, Down's syndrome

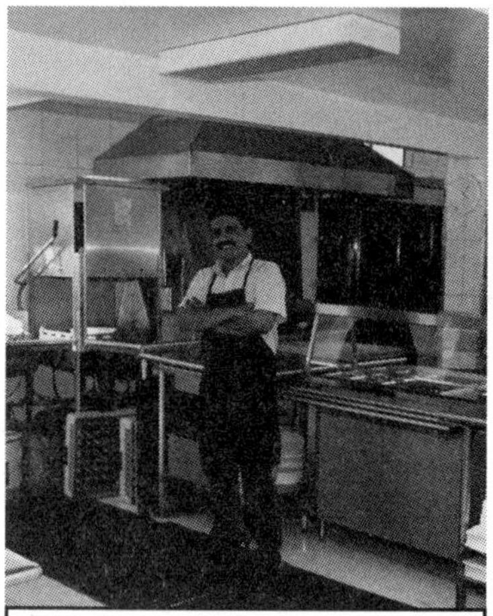

Kitchen

Dr. Robert Bradford

Dr. Bradford is president of American Biologics and the Bradford Research Institute and is the holder of nine patents and two honorary doctorates. He has authored many publications including a co-authorship of the very profound International Protocols for Individualized, Integrated Metabolic Programs in Cancer Management.

Dr. Robert Bradford is one of the world's major pioneers in the research, development and application of metabolic/nutritional therapy. He gave up a scientific career as a consultant and technical staff member of Stanford University, California, to lead one of the greatest crusades in modern times, which is no less than a medical revolution and a political reformation.

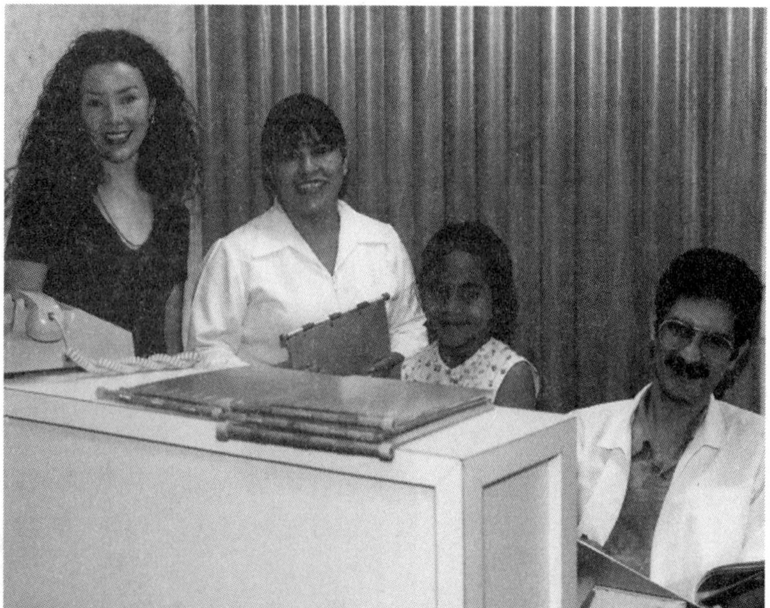

American Biologics' Hospital Staff

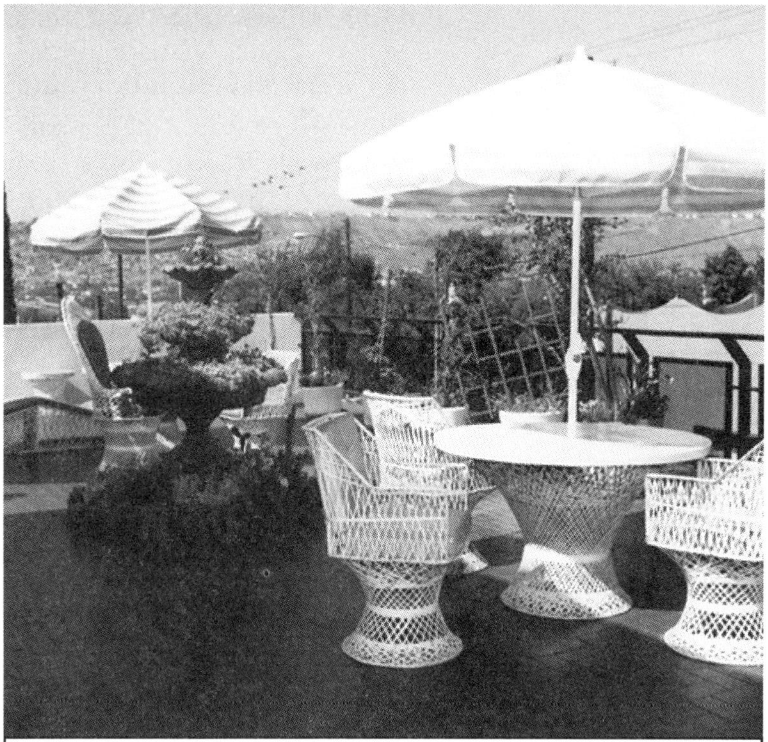

Patio Area

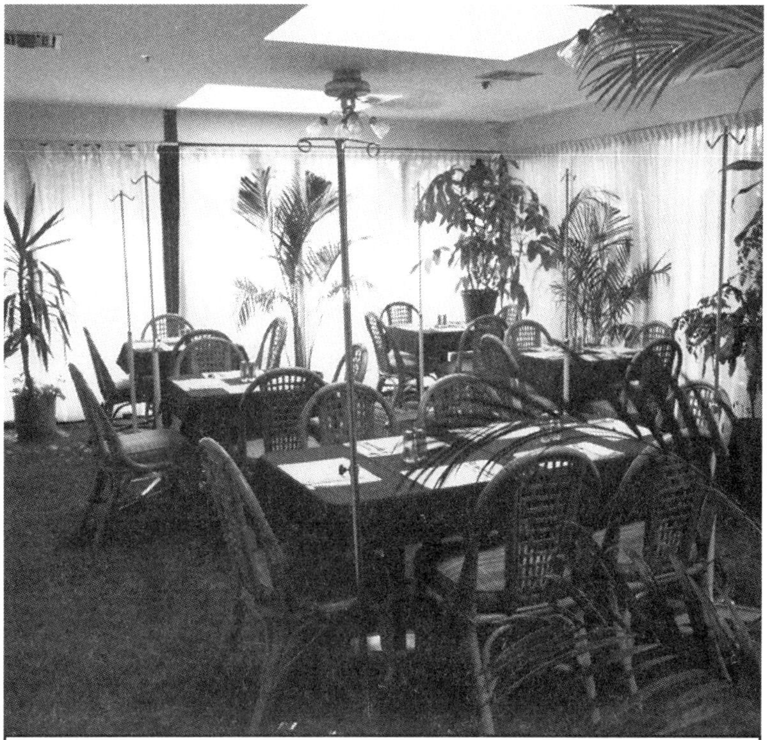

Dining Room

American Metabolic Institute

American Metabolic Institute,
420 Granados FRACC La Mesa, Tijuana, B.C. Mexico
For mailing: 555 Saturn Boulevard Building B, M/S432
San Diego, CA 92154
(800) 388-1083
(619) 267-1107
(619) 229-3003
Fax: (619)267-1109
011-52-66-217602
011-52-66-217603

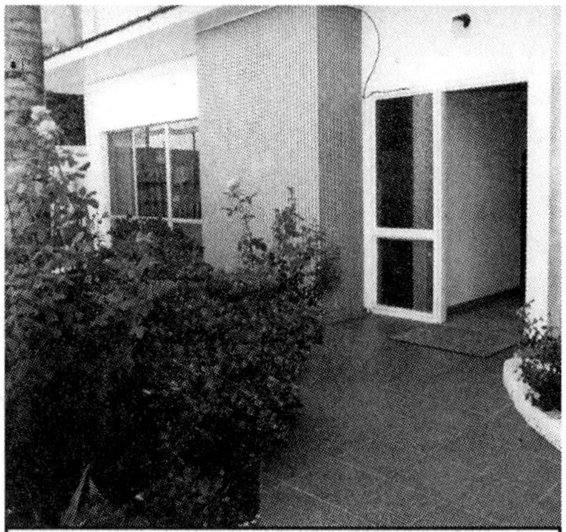

American Metabolic Institute

American Metabolic Institute (A.M.I.) and the St. Joseph Hospital are located four miles south of the San Diego border.

The facility resides in a temperate climate surrounded by flower gardens and palm trees plus swimming pool.

The A.M.I. program is focused on holistic healing of body, mind and spirit. Every patient is given an individualized metabolic program to follow which includes tests, detoxification, a catabolic diet and pH balancing. Preparation for the program begins with a series of non-invasive tests given to determine severity of disease, then ongoing tests throughout therapy to determine efficacy of treatment. They include blood toxicology tests, live cell analysis, iridology examination as well as regular blood and urine tests. Kinesiology

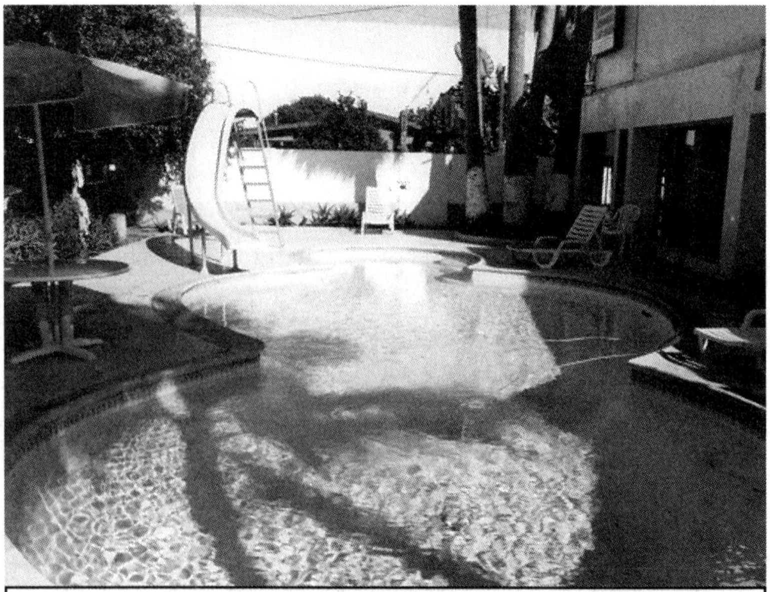

Pool Area

(muscle testing) is given for possible allergic reaction to supplements. Diagnostic X-rays are sometimes recommended.

Fasting, colonics and lymphatic massage is given to help detoxify the colon, kidneys, skin and lungs. Coffee enemas are used to relieve the edema that occurs with some kinds of cancers.

The catabolic diet consists of cancer fighting organic foods, juices and herbal teas such as red clover, chaparral and Pau de Arco.

Balancing pH is accomplished with the use of diet and immune enhancing therapies. Therapies most used at A.M.I. Clinic and Hospital are Laetrile, vitamin A, enzymes, amino acids, Rodaquin, Glymyd, DMSO, growth hormone therapy, germanium, clodronate immune-enhancing vaccines, homeopathic medicines, external herbal creams, and chelation.

Because cancer rotates RNA and DNA to the right, much care is given to the quality of medicines, their use and strength and their rotation to the left to insure healing.

A.M.I. specializes in using various kinds of herbal formulas for various kinds of cancers. An in-house herbal pharmacy permits individualization of formulas and immediate adjustments as patient requirements change.

Estrogen blockers and non-toxic chemotherapy called Flutamid are sometimes used. Surgery and/or low-dose radiation may be used in special cases.

Some additional services provided are acupuncture, chiropractic and reflexology.

- Specialty: detoxification program, regeneration, breast, and skin

American Metabolic Institute has a full hospital staff of doctors, nurses and therapists.

The Institute is also known for being one of the first in the Americas to use Bio-electric Medicine and will probably gain future recognition for being another first for the revival and successful use of the Rife (frequency machine) and other Bio-Magnetic Therapies (including the use of SE5-MDR). Bill Fry has been in the forefront of A.MAI.'s Bio-electric Medicine.

The A.M.I. Facility provides both in-patient and out-patient services. The average cost for a three week stay is about $7,000 for cancer therapy. Preventative programs are available for about $1,400 a week. Some American insurances and credit cards are accepted.

American Metabolic Institute has a full hospital staff of doctors nurses and therapists. Dr. Rubio, is well known and respected by his peers for his successful use of autogenous vaccines. He is one of the first doctors to make vaccines from tumor tissues. He is a Medical Director of American Metabolic Institute.

Dr. Geronimo Rubio, M.D.

Dr. Geronimo Rubio, M.D. received his M.D. degree from the University if Autonoma de Baja California Medical school in Mexico. Through his studies at the University he did research in the Departments of Physiology, Biochemistry, Bacteriology and Parasitology. He discovered that flowers brought into the hospital rooms were infecting patients with bacteria strains of Pseudomonad Aure Ginosa.

For the last 9 years, he has researched and developed a process of RNA transference in lymphocytes, polypeptide formulas for cancer cells and developed the formula for the blocking factors in tumor cells.

William Fry

William Fry attended the University of Phoenix, Arizona, majoring in Business Administration. He has worked in the fields in the fields of Engineering Documentation and researching the health field for over 20 years. He is also a Medical Director of American Metabolic Institute.

Mr. Fry introduced the Royal Rife Frequency Generator technology to Mexico. He has developed protocols for various diseases using the Rife Generator.

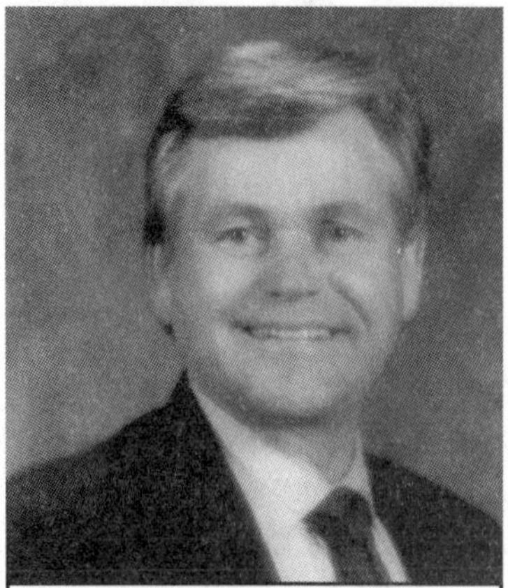

William Fry

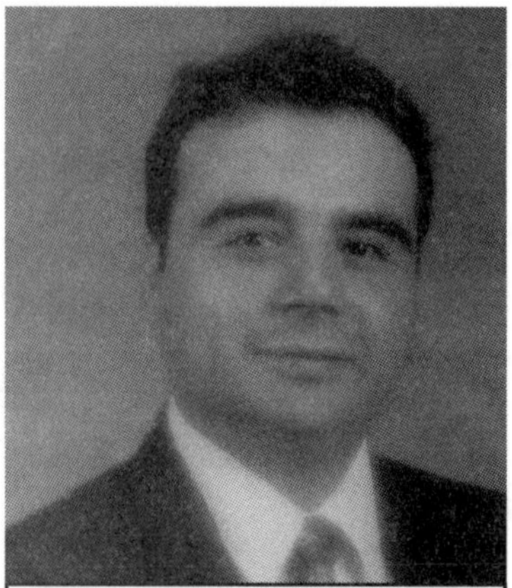

Dr. Geronimo Rubio, M.D.

Bio-Medical Center (Hoxsey Therapy)

615 General Ferreira (Colonia Juarez)
Tijuana, B.C. Mexico
For mailing: P.O. Box 727 Tijuana, B.C. Mexico
011-52-84-9011
Evenings: 011-52-814-9132

The Hoxsey treatment was named after John Hoxsey, who in 1840 formulated three herbal formulas.

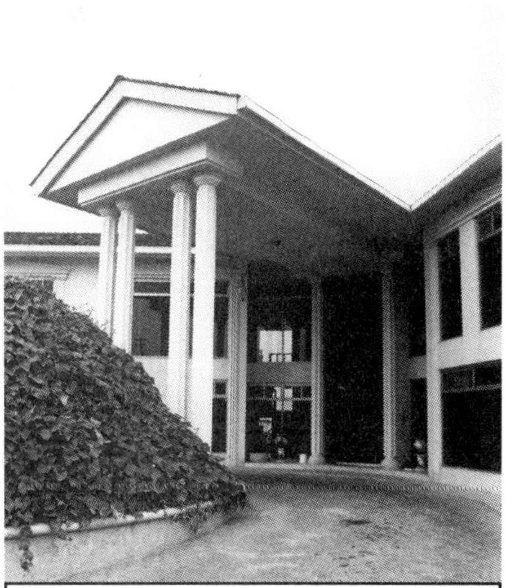

Bio-Medical Clinic

John made the discovery of the herbs because one of his horses had a cancerous sore on his leg. Not having the heart to shoot the horse, John him put out to pasture. The sore on the horse's leg began to dry up and peel off. John discovered the horse had found an area of the farm that was rich in vegetation and herbs. The horse was eating the herbs and putting some of the masticated herbs on his sore leg. John examined all of the herbs very carefully. He ground them, soaked them, juiced them and he came up with three formulas: one that is used internally that looks like black cough syrup, and two that are used externally, a yellow powder and a red paste. The internal formula consists of licorice, red clover, burdock root, stillingia root, berberis root, poke root, cascara amarga, prickly ash bark, buckthorn bark and potassium iodine. The yellow powder contain escharotic agents that have been known since ancient times for the treatment of external cancers. They are suphide, yellow precipitate, sulphur and talc. The red paste is made of antimony trisulphide, zinc chloride and bloodroot. The formula used internally helps to balance the acid/alkaline of the body and deals with the DNA, bringing it back to a more normal state. The external formulas dry the sores and they come off.

These formulas were first used on John Hoxsey's horses and then on family members and friends. The formulas were handed down to John's grandson, Harry Hoxsey.

Each generation was told to protect the formula and to treat anyone who came to them even if they couldn't pay and to remember that treating people is a duty and a privilege.

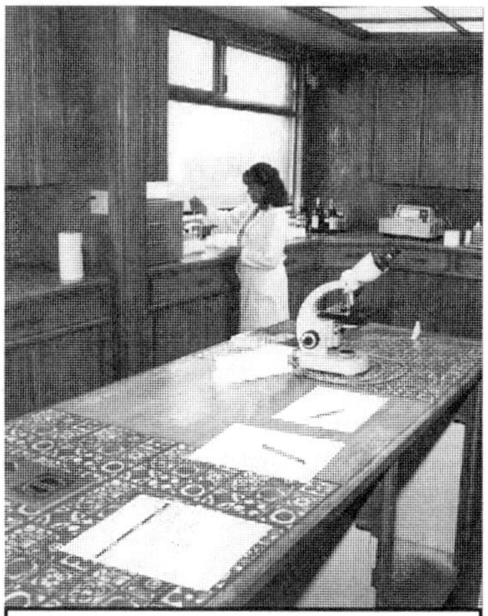

Laboratory

After the death of Harry Hoxsey in 1973, Mildred Nelson, a registered nurse, became the owner and director of the Hoxsey Clinic. Mildred first came to the clinic with her mother who had cancer. Harry asked her, "Mildred, you are a nurse, why don't you come and work for me?" Mildred told Dr. Hoxsey, "I think you are a quack. I have come here only upon the request of my mother." Then Harry said to her, "If I cure your mother, will you come and work for me?" Mildred answered, "If you cure my mother, I'll work for you the rest of my life." And so it is that 41 years later, Mildred's mother is still okay today.

The Hoxsey Out-patient Clinic was first located in Dallas, Texas. In 1963, Dr. Hoxsey moved the clinic to Tijuana, Mexico, where it is located today. Five doctors are employed at the clinic. Patients who arrive early (before 9:00 a.m.) are seen Monday through Friday without an appointment. They are given a complete work-up: a

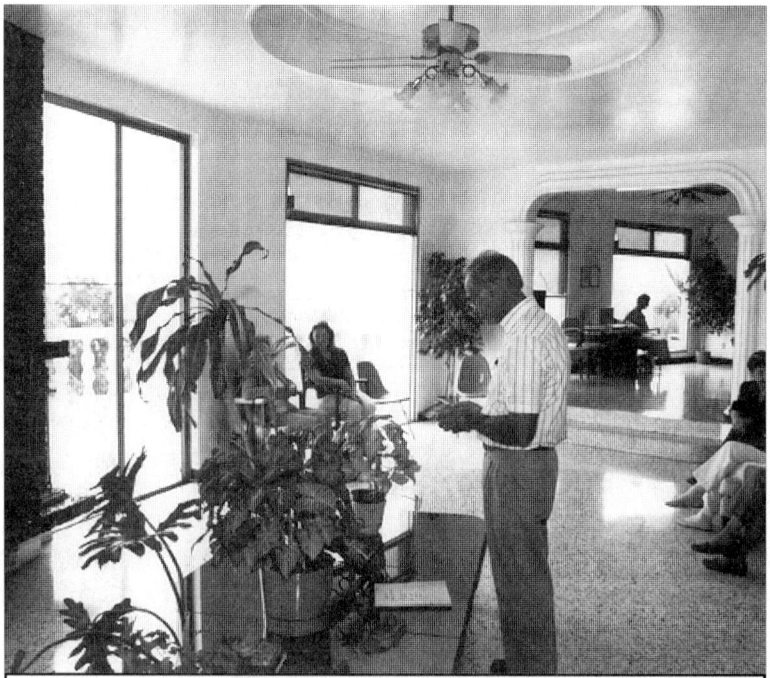

Patient Waiting Room

physical examination, lab work, X-rays and a clinical history is taken. They are advised to bring any other medical records from other hospitals or facilities. After their one-day appointment, they return home with enough vitamins and Hoxsey formula to last several months. The total cost of the Hoxsey treatment is $3,500 for the term of the illness. Patients can return at any time as long as they are following the prescribed treatment.

- Specialty: skin cancer, emphysema, kidney and stomach disorders, lungs, acute and chronic leukemia

Mildred Nelson, R.N.

"I'm just a dumb nurse," says Mildred Nelson, ". . . if I'd been smart, I'd have been a doctor." For more than 40 years, Mildred has treated more cancer patients than all the other Tijuana clinics combined. John Hoxsey's grandson, Harry, made no mistake when he entrusted this lady to protect his grandfather's special formula. As a result, the Hoxsey tonic has remained the same original formula without any changes or alterations of its ingredients, strength or preparation. In addition, Mildred has proven the John Hoxsey formula to be more than just common "horse sense" (first used on John's horses). She has done this, not with laboratory mice, but with literally thousands of patients who attest to the efficacy and validity of its benefits. Long standing, consistent and persistent, the Hoxsey Therapy continues as word of mouth brings more and more patients to the clinic. Although Miss Nelson has always invited any honest investigation of her patients' files, the AMA has been more interested in the ingredients of the formula rather than how it works on human beings. As a result of the AMA's not really wanting to know, Mildred has found that her time is better spent getting results than trying to prove them.

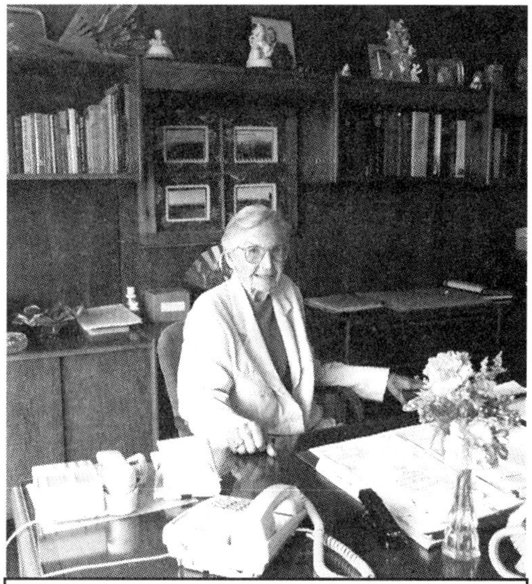

Mildred Nelson

Biological Medicine Institute

Avenida de la Paz #16420 Colonia Mineral Sante Fe
Tijuana, B.C. 22360 Mexico
For mailing: P.O. Box 433656
San Ysidro, California 92173
011-52-66-240786
011-52-66-240939
011-52-66-245110

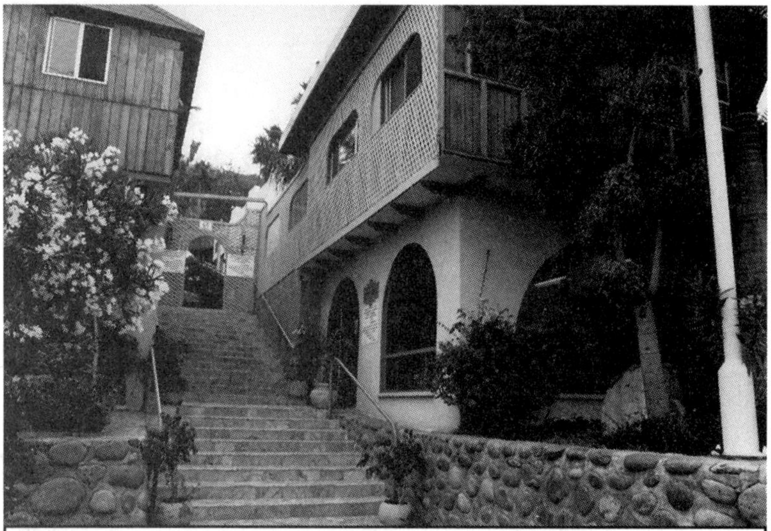

Biological Medicine Institute

The Biological Medicine Institute (Institute de Medincina Biologica) is located in the complex of the beautiful Agua Termales

Valparaiso has Tijuana's only natural running sulfur hot springs. Dr. Harvey Bigleson is director of the institute. Learning much from the history of famous doctors, their achievements and their errors, Dr. Harvey Bigelson states, "I have cast my lot with Hahnemann, Bechamp and Enderlein. The pleomorphic doctrine is a true one. It works. We are a body of germs. They live with us in harmony when we are healthy, but there is the potential for them to become harmful if the terrain breaks down. I see it every day, because I study live blood. I use a darkfield microscope which magnifies 1200 times."

"Probably one of the most dramatic things I've seen is the growth of cancer in a drop of fresh blood. If the blood dies on the slide in two hours, that patient, whose blood it is, is very sick. If the blood lives on the slide for five days, the donor is healthy. In a cancer, the darkfield analysis actually shows mold growing as the blood loses its nutrition, its oxygen."

"One of the most satisfying experiences is when I can see on a darkfield analysis the blood of a cancer patient returning to form. I know the patient is improving and that pleomorphism has been vindicated."

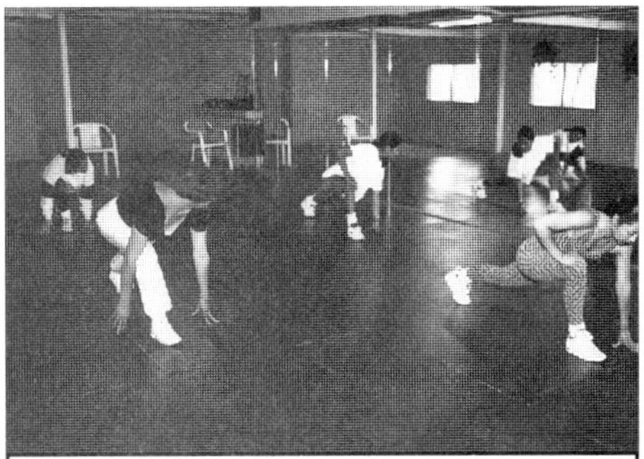

Aerobics Class

Dr. Bigelson believes, as do Royal Rife and Virginia Livingston Wheeler, that fungi, bacteria and virus change in form, confirming what Bechamp observed 100 years earlier. "Cancer is a mold of the human body and it takes years to get there. The average cancer is present 39 months before the patient even knows it and the doctor can detect it. It makes no difference if there is one spot or a hundred spots of metastasis, if the mold is eliminated in one place it will be eliminated in all hundred places."

"Germs don't cause disease, they live in a diseased environment."

"The terrain that leads to the disease of cancer is one that is anaerobic alkaline. A reading of 7.2 ½-alkaline and over is the time for prevention, before the terrain leads to disease."

"In using biological therapies based on the pleomorphic concept, we bring back the pH to a state of normalcy. When the pH is changed, the terrain is changed—detoxified."

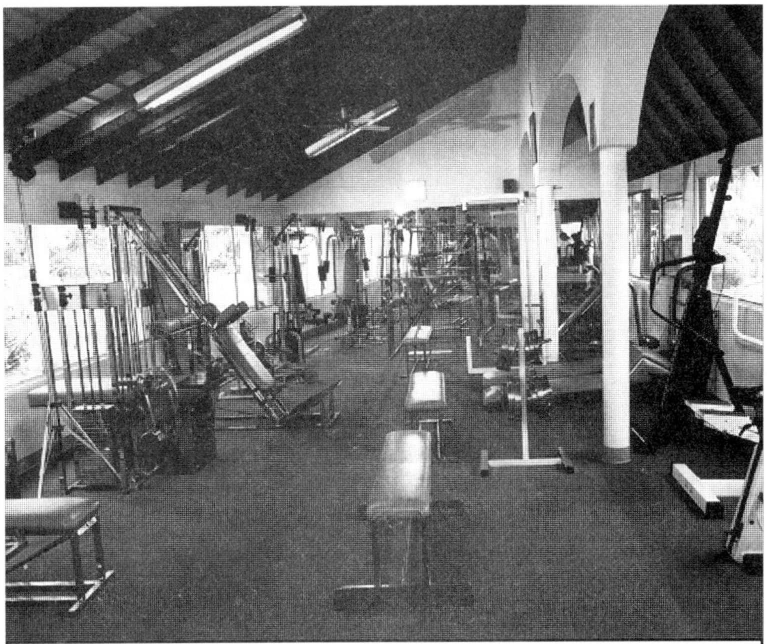

Weight Room

"We use homeopathy and biological remedies. The goad of Homeopathy is not to "kill" germs, viruses and bacteria, but to strengthen the whole body and enhance the immune system. The body must be allowed to cure in the way it wants, not the way of the physician."

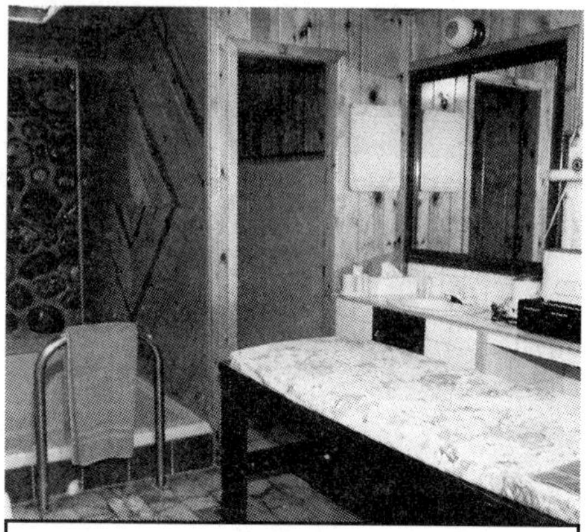

Private Spa

"The diet of the cancer patient is very important. The germ and the host have to be kept happy with nutrition. Most cancer patients don't die of cancer, but of malnutrition, because the cancer is robbing them of nitrogen. And because cancer feeds on nitrogen, potassium, calcium and iron, diets have to be regulated to prevent feeding the cancers."

Emotional counseling at the Institute is always taken into consideration. It has now been seen through Magnetic Resonance Imaging that there is activity in the brain, accompanying emotion. Moods and attitudes do physically affect the tissues and the organs of the body and the immune system.

Cosmetic services are also available at the Institute using growth hormone extracts. Biological Medicine Institute offers in-patient accommodations for those desiring to stay in Tijuana. The Agua Termales Valparaiso offers motel and restaurant services.

Prices at the Institute range from $2,500 to $3,500 a week for cancer therapy.

- Specialty: Alzheimer's, heart, circulatory

Harvey Bigelson, M.D.

Some excerpts from Health Freedom News, June, 1993. Dr. Harvey Bigelson with Janet Stoeppelmann (with permission).

Harvey Bigelson, M.D. was born in Brooklyn, New York. He attended Kenyon College, Gambier, Ohio; State University, Buffalo, New York; and Buffalo School of Medicine. He completed his internship in Pasadena, California and received his Medical Degree in 1965. In 1969, after three years of Ophthalmology residency in Buffalo, New York, he was drafted into the Army and sent to Vietnam. There he headed an Emergency Room

Trauma Unit and was honorably discharged in 1970 with the rank of major.

In 1971, Dr Bigleson started his own Ophthalmology practice in Princeton, New Jersey and later became interested in homeopathy. He worked at the ARE clinic in Phoenix, Arizona and soon opened his own holistic practice in Phoenix in 1978. He became the state coordinator for the American Holistic Medical Association.

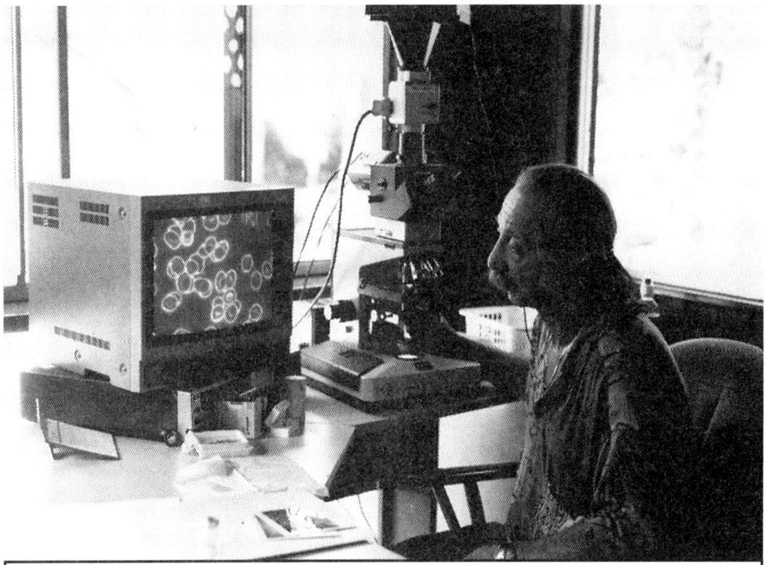

Harvey Bigelson, M.D.

In 1981 he was appointed President of Arizona's Board of Homeopathic Medicine Examiners (HOMEX) by Governor Bruce Babbitt.

In 1981 he was appointed president of Arizona's Board of Homeopathic Medicine Examiners (HOMEX) by Governor Bruce Babbitt. Dr. Bigelson drafted the most encompassing standards and laws for the practice of homeopathy and alternative medicine in the United States, and in 1981 he founded the Arizona Homeopathic Medical Association. In 1986 he was sponsored to study in Germany the Dr. Guenther Enderlein's medical theories. He returned to his own private homeopathic practice at his clinic, the Center for Progressive Medicine in Scottsdale, Arizona. He is presently practicing in Tijuana, Mexico with offices located within the complex of the beautiful Agua Termales Valparaiso.

Dr. Bigelson is also conducting a study in conjunction with seven other United States universities using LK-200 which is a multiple cocktail of human interferon and interlukins. He has exclusive use of the product in Tijuana.

Castillo Clinic

The Castillo Clinic has its own dental office.
Dr. Silva Palacios Roji is the Clinic's on staff dentist.
Jose Gorostiza 1121-2 Zona Rio Tijuana, B.C. Mexico
For Mailing: 416 W. San Yisdro Blvd. #L-337
San Ysidro, CA 92173
011-52-66-835700
011-52-66-835701
011-52-66-836016

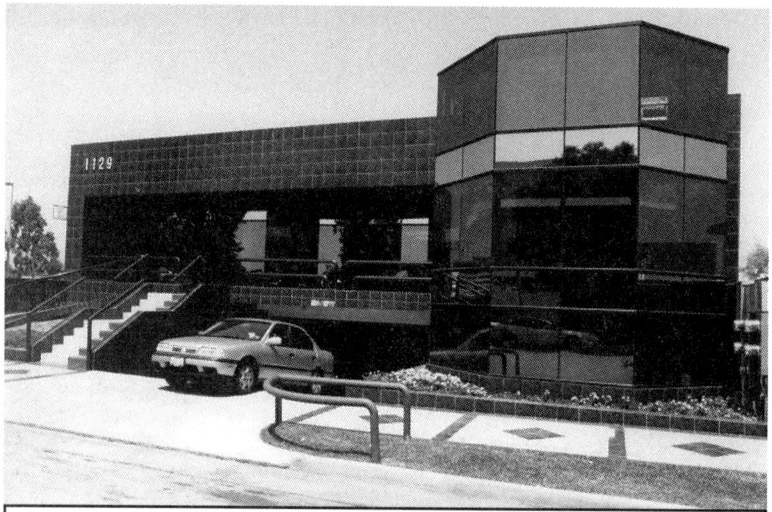

Castillo Clinic

The Castillo Clinic is well known for its expert use of chelation therapy and for integrating therapies from around the world.

Most forms of cancer are treated at the clinic, as well as arthritis, vascular disorders (heart attack, strokes, high blood pressure), toxicities, immune-related diseases, deterioration attributed to the aging process, and premature aging.

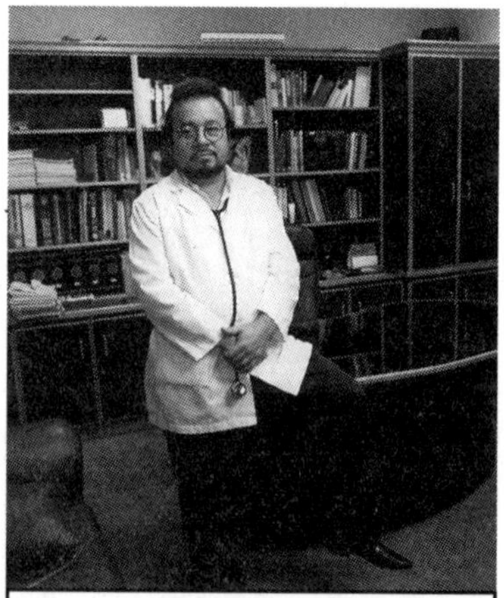

Dr. Castillo

Dr. Castillo states, "Diseases start out silently. The cues of the body breaking down are very vague and often go undetected until disease has progressed to the degree that symptoms and disease are apparent."

"We treat sick people, not disease. We do this by teaching people to detect important initial signs that indicate the beginning of disease, such as in the deterioration of the nervous system; a person may show signs of memory loss, or poor reflexes.

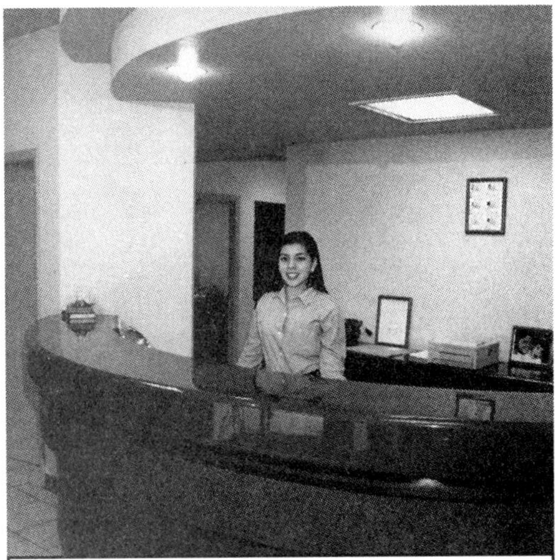
Reception Desk

Dry scaling skin may be a sign of a deteriorating circulatory system. Weakness in extremities may be a cue that the skeletal system is breaking down. Hyperactivity or sluggishness may point to the endocrine system."

"In all cases, we treat the causes of diseases, as well as the symptoms." Treatment at the Castillo Clinic consists of chelation therapy, Laetrile, growth hormone therapy, Hoxsey treatment and hydrogen peroxide.

Chelation is used for: 1) obstruction of circulation (hardening of arteries); 2) abnormal calcium deposits (as in arthritis, bursitis, tendonitis, bone spurs and osteoporosis); and 3) toxicities (drugs, alcohol, heavy metals). Laetrile is used as an anti-tumor agent.

Growth hormone (mammal tissue) is used from various organs to treat cancer, diabetes, M.S., amyotrophic lateral sclerosis (Lou Gehrig's Disease), lupus E, cerebral palsy, Down's Syndrome, autism, spinal afflictions, osteoporosis, chronic hepatitis, asthma, bronchitis, rheumatism, sterility, impotence, Parkinson's Disease, and general degeneration of the immune system.

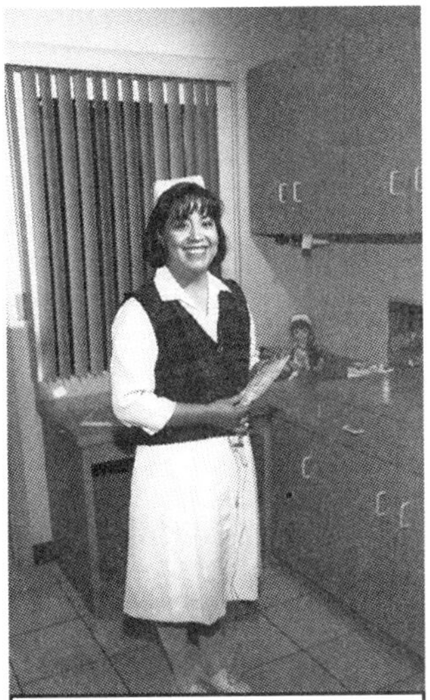
Nurses Station

The herbal Hoxsey tonic, a blend of herbs and potassium, is used to help detoxify and cleanse the liver and blood. Hydrogen peroxide is used like an antibiotic and oxygenator to help kill bacteria, viruses, and other parasites associated with malignancies.

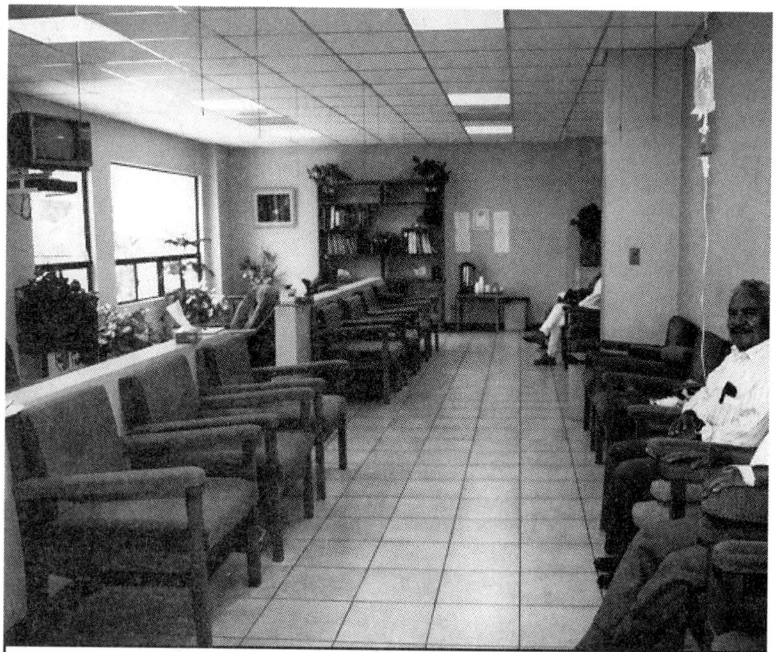

Patient Chelation and Nutrition I.V. Room

Prevention is emphasized at the Castillo Clinic, along with the importance of maintaining good health by periodic testing and a continuing maintenance program after the completion of primary treatments.

Dr. Yolanda Fraire is part of the Castillo Clinic staff and is in charge of Homeopathic Medicine.

Prevention is emphasized at the Castillo Clinic.

The removal of silver—mercury fillings plays a major role in the medical treatment of heart and cancer patients. The Castillo Clinic has its own dental office.

Dr. Silva Palacios Roji is the Clinic's on staff dentist.

- Specialities: arteriosclerosis, diabetes, multiple sclerosis, amyotrophic lateral sclerosis (Lou Gehrig's Disease), lupus

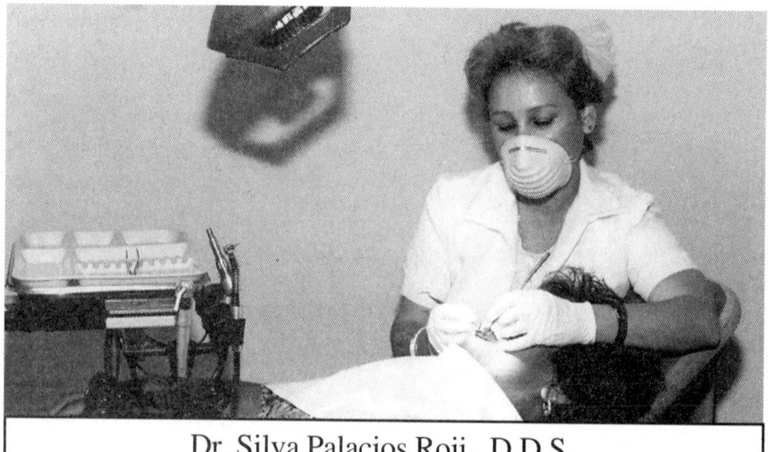

Dr. Silva Palacios Roji , D.D.S.

Contreras' Metabolic Therapy

Hospital Ernesto Contreras
Paseo de Tijuana 1-A Playas de Tijuana, Mexico
For mailing: 2505 Congress Street, Suite 120
San Diego, CA 92110
(800) 700-1850
011-52-66-801850
Fax: 011-52-66-801855

There are several clinics in Tijuana, Mexico, but the Ernesto Contreras Hospital and clinic is probably the most famous for being the first to use Laetrile in the treatment of cancer.

Dr. Contreras is the founder and Medical Director of the hospital and clinic. Dr. Contreras has over 40 years' experience treating cancer patients (over 50,000) with Amygdalin (Laetrile) and other non-toxic metabolic therapies. Laetrile is the basic anti-tumor agent used at the Contreras Hospital and Clinic, and they are proud of using a Laetrile produced by KEM, S.A. Laboratories (Kemdalin) as it is of the highest quality and strictly controlled by a scientific board.

Dr. Contreras treats his patients holistically—body, mind and spirit—and believes that someday there will be professionally trained people, ministers, who are oncologists, and psychiatrists who are oncologists who will be a part of every cancer patient's treatment program. He counsels his patients for any emotional problems they may be having and believes that stress is a major factor in the cause of disease. "Sometimes we have seen tumors disappear in three or four days and we have not done anything except to give that person psychotherapy or counselng. Their own natural interferon has started to heal them." Dr. Contreras also has his own church where non-denominational services are held for his patients.

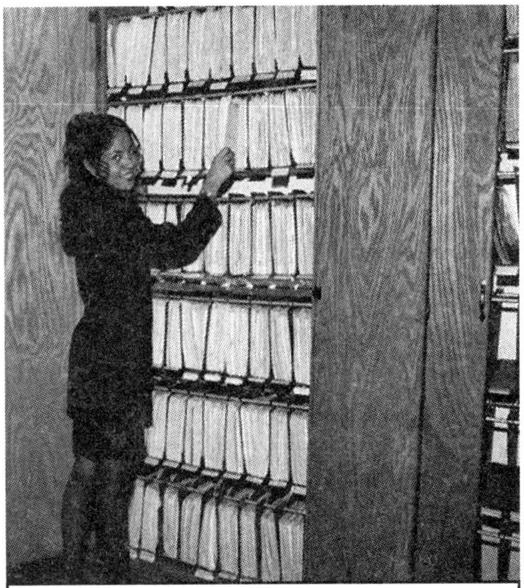

Medical Records

When treating the patient biologically, Dr. Contreras treats the host (body) as well as the parasite (cancer) as do most of the non-toxic cancer clinics. This is done with the use of proteolytic enzymes, megadoses of vitamins A and C, multi-vitamins and minerals, immunology, Laetrile, stress reduction programs, detoxification and detoxifiation diet.

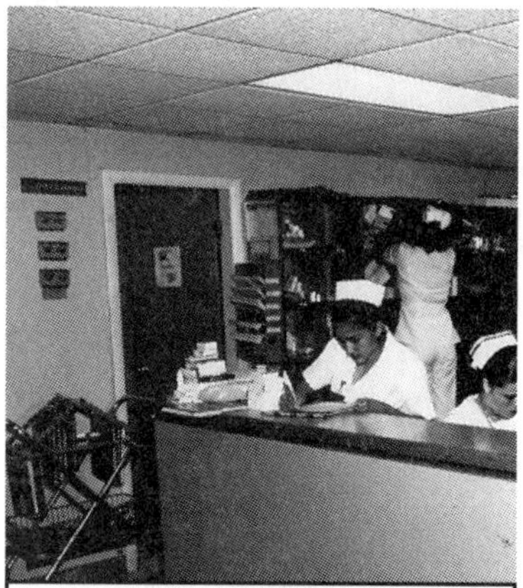

Nurses Station

Preventive medicine that is also practiced at the Contreras Hospital for early detection of cancer (precancerous condition before it becomes a tumor) and other chronic diseases is available for anyone. Blood tests (AMID, CEA) and urine tests (Navarro, protein) may be used for this purpose. Relatives and friends of the patients are welcome to use these services. Remember: One day of prevention is far better than a lifetime of treatments. This day of testing is usually less than $300.

The hospital complex also includes a restaurant with a Laetrile diet and the Girosoles Motel and Trailer Park. Transportation to and from San Diego Airport is available upon request.

The cost for treatment at Hospital Ernesto Contreras is approximately $8,000 to $11,000 for a three week stay.

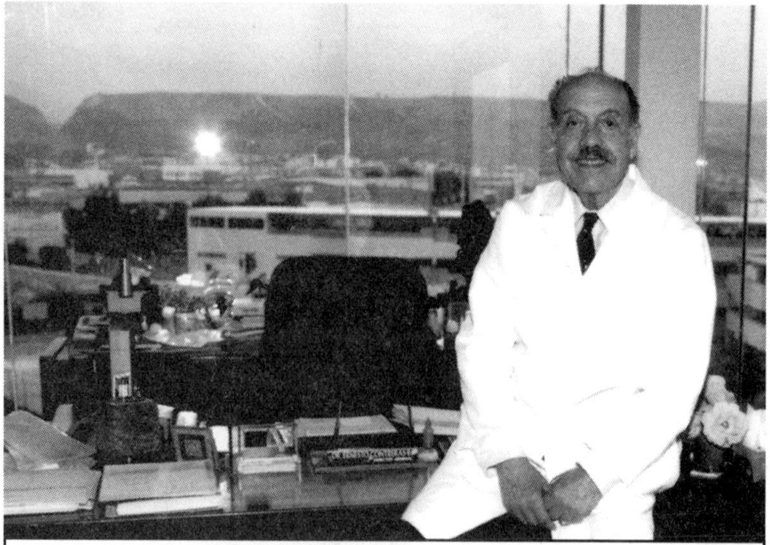

Dr. Ernesto Contreras, Sr.

- Specialty: breast lymphoma, prostate, leukemia, colon, lung

Ernesto Contreras, M.D.

Dr. Contreras is a graduate of the Army Medicine School in Mexico City. His postgraduate studies were at the Children's Hospital in Boston, Massachusetts.

Ernesto Contreras, M.D., pathologist and oncologist, is famous for his pioneer work with Laetrile. He was born in Guadalajara, Jal., Mexico, in 1915. He graduated as physician and surgeon in 1939. After working as a general practitioner from 1940 to 1943, he then specialized in hematology and pathology.

Dr. Contreras founded the Del Mar Medical Center and Hospital in 1970 and is presently the Medical Director and Chief Oncologist.

Dr. Contreras became Subchief Pathologist of Army General Hospital, Mexico City, 1944-1953; Subchief Pathologist of Children's Hospital, 1944-1955, Boston, MA; Chief Pathologist Army General Hospital, 1953-1955; Chief Pathologist Pasteur Laboratories, Tijuana, B.C., 1955-1957; Associate Pathologist Mercy Hospital, San Diego, CA, 1959-1964; and he was organizer of the First Early Detection Cancer Center in Baja California, Mexico.

Dr. Contreras is the founder and active member of both the National College of Army Doctors and the Mexican Association of Oncology Studies since 1954. He holds active membership in the following: Mexican Association of Pathology; Latin American Association of Pathology; World Medical Association; International Union Against Cancer; Sonora-Baja California Federation of Medical Doctors. He has been the author of several publications which include the Phase I, Phase II and Phase III Clinical Studies on Amygdalin and Phase III Study on Inoperable Cancer of the Lung. He has been using metabolic therapy, including Laetrile, since 1965.

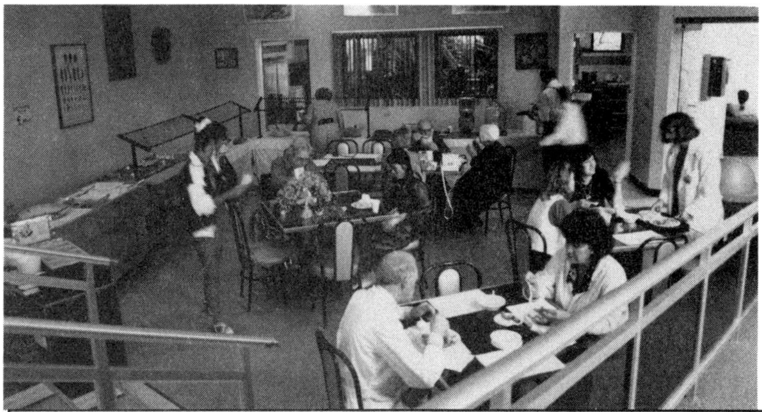

Buffet Dining Room

Genesis West Provida (Organo Therapy)

Calle Roga #1340 SECC Jardines, FRACC
Playas de Tijuana, Baja, Mexico 22700
For mailing: P.O. Box 3460
Chula Vista, CA 91909
(619) 424-9552
011-52-66-301313
011-52-66-802528

Instutito Genesis West Provida is located near Tijuana in Playas only a few blocks from the beach.

Genesis West Provida specializes in rehabilitation programs before and after chemotherapy, radiation, and surgery. They do this with programs using biological medicine therapies.

Biological medicine therapies consist of biological response modifiers and vaccines, organo or growth hormone therapy, bio-energetic medicine (which includes the myopulse and electro-acuscope), short-wave hyperthermia, detoxification dietary programs, ozone hydrotherapy, homeopathies, nutritional and herbal supplementation.

Genesis prides itself on in its organo therapy which helps the individual organs to regenerate themselves. Organo therapy helps to regenerate the whole body.

Initially, the patient taking the organo therapy will experience minimal, if any, reactions from this specialized therapy. However, after about six to twelve

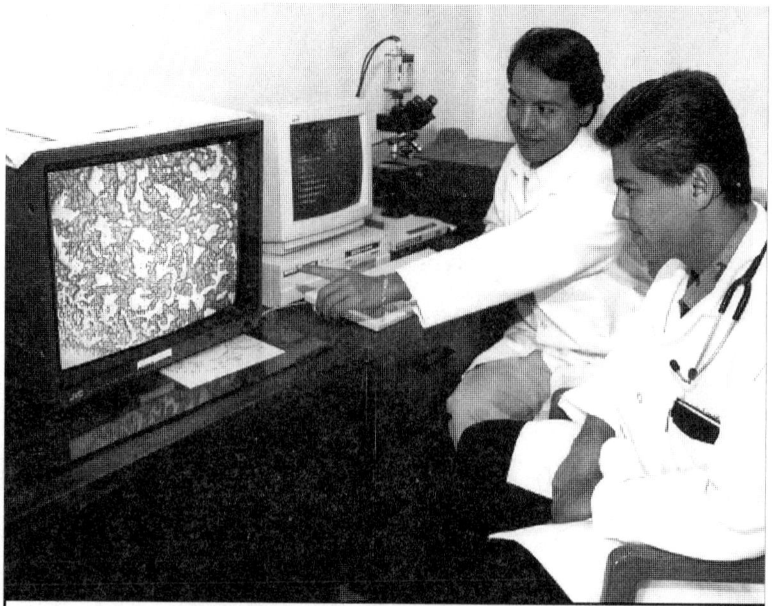

Cell Analysis With Darkfield Microscope

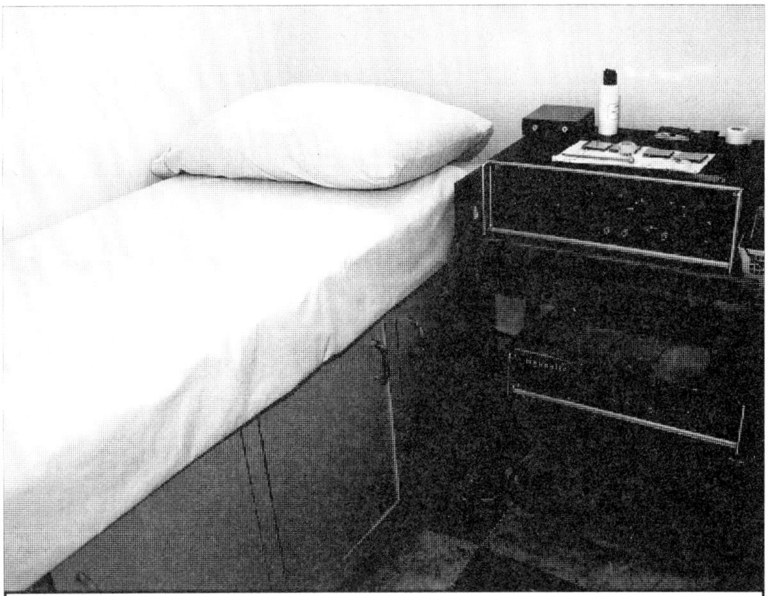

Acuscope Machine

weeks following therapy, the following changes are expected to occur: The joints and discs will become more flexible, weight will tend to stabilize at a normal level, and vigor will replace previous lethargy. A new willingness and desire to experience life and its rewards will emerge, as will the desire to initiate new enterprises. There will be renewed sexual satisfaction, and generally an enthusiastic appetite to become more involved with life. Also during that same time, the individual will begin to look more youthful and alive. This is projected not only from inside the body, but outside as well, as eyes clear and skin tone, texture and color improve. Genesis feels that treating their clients holistically with growth hormone therapy is better than treating symptoms.

Some of the other modalities offered at Genesis West are: A detoxification program geared toward the client's individual problem, colonics, massage, sauna, herbal baths, special exercise, mind and stress therapy, chelation, DMSO and Laetrile.

Some of the tests provided at the clinic are: SMA 24, CBC, urinalysis, Darkfield including clot retraction microscope re-evaluation of subcellular systems. A pap smear for women or hair analysis are available if recommended.

Bio-energetic evaluations include synchrodyne 520 tests and electro-acuscope evaluation. Consultant services are also available such as X-ray, surgery, skin specialists, biological dentist, etc.

At West Provida Clinic, a team of medical professionals have years of experience in the field of growth hormone therapy and clients feel confident coming to West because of their expertise in the field.

Andrew McNaughton is the research consultant. Andrew is a pioneer in the field of holistic and metabolic medications and practices and has, in the past, helped many of the other alternative clinics research their best therapies. On staff are Drs. Amerscau and Videl.

West Provida's director and administrator is Jacob Swilling, Ph.D.

The cost of therapy at Genesis West is approximately $3800 per week and may vary according to individual therapy.

- Specialty: rejuvenation, skin

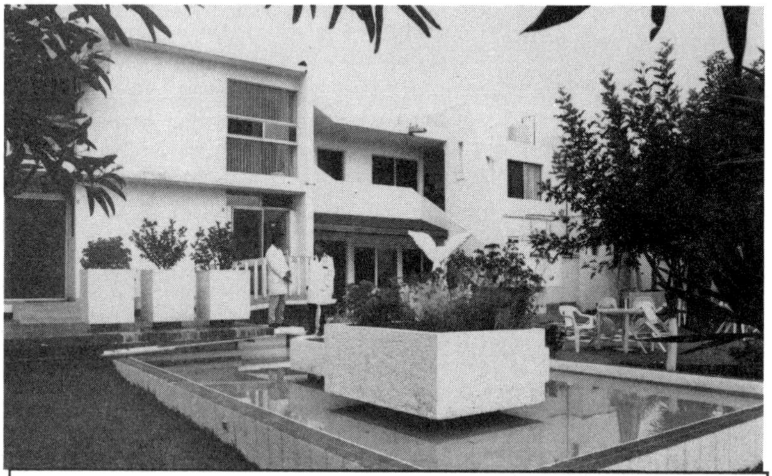

Yard & Patio Area

Andrew McNaughton

Andrew McNaughton's education includes degrees in business, electrical and aeronautical engineering, geology and mining, and a four year classical course under the Jesuits at Loyola College in Montreal, Canada. He served in the Royal Canadian Air Force from 1939 to 1946 and was awarded the Air Force Cross for his work as a test pilot. He is a member of the Canadian Aeronautics and Space Institute, the Canadian's Test Pilots' Association, the New York Academy of Sciences, the Executive Board of the Institute of Nutritional Research, and the John Beard Research Institute. In 1968 he became a Knight of the Order of the Hospital of Saint John of Jerusalem (Malta), Grand Priory of Dacia. In 1970 he was appointed a Member of the Court of Benefactors of the Royal Society of Medicine in England.

The Gerson Clinic

(Gerson Institute) at CHIPSA
446 Nubes Playas De Tijuana
For mailing: P.O. Box 430 Bonita, CA 91908
Info packets and books: (619) 472-7450

The Gerson Therapy is probably best known for its special diet which includes a lot of carrot juice and the use of coffee enemas. Dr. Gerson learned of using the coffee enemas during World War I when they were used to reduce pain when morphine was not available. He had also read that tests had proven this to work on animals. Realizing the levels of toxin was reduced, he later used the coffee enemas in his therapy along with a special diet.

Dr. Gerson's special diet was one that he had discovered for himself when he was just out of medical school.

He suffered from mi-graine head-aches, making it almost impossible to practice, and the medical books gave no cure for them. He started using one food at a time. At first he tried milk which was a complete failure. He then looked to the pri-mates and de-cided to try apples. With the apples he found success and then added and subtracted foods according to his tolerance.

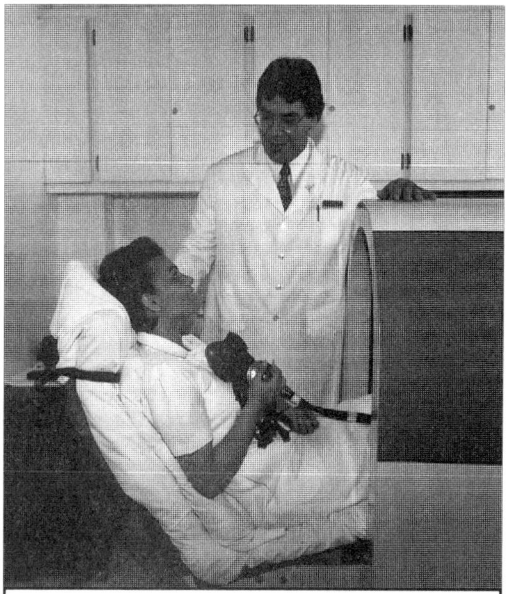
Hyberbaric Oxygen Chamber

One day a patient arrived in his office with migraines. Dr. Gerson explained to him that the books say there is no cure for your headaches, but this is what I do. The patient tried Dr. Gerson's diet and was successful in getting rid of his migraines also.

Another patient came to him with migraines and was relieved not only of his migraines, but of his lupus as well. This patient sent to Dr. Gerson several other lupus patients and he treated and cured them. Dr. Gerson was brought before the courts in Germany by physicians complaining that he was not a skin specialist. But because there wasn't anyone else in the court that could cure lupus, the judge said, "Then let this man do it."

Dr. Gerson prescribed his diet and enemas to many patients and with success they recovered from different illnesses. Later, having heard of his success, a lady came to him who had cancer. He told her that he didn't know anything about treating cancer, that it was different. She told him that she would sign a paper releasing him of all responsibility if he would only treat her. She survived and he then began to receive other cancer patients that had heard of his success in treating cancer.

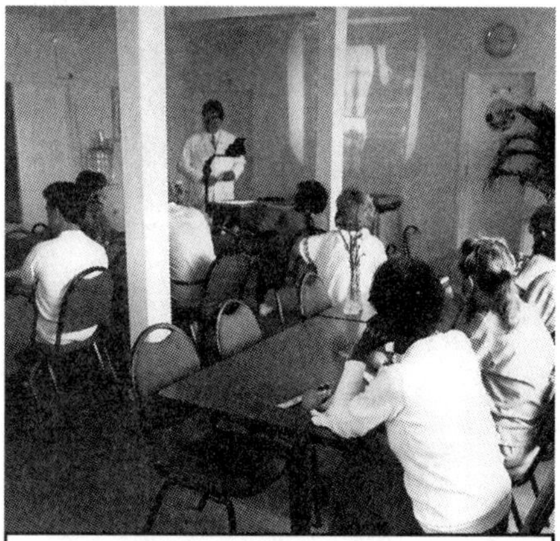

Patient Training Room

In the beginning, Dr. Gerson had not always been successful with all of his patients and he blamed his failures upon certain foods. Over the years he made many changes before he perfected his diet. Today this special diet, the Gerson Diet, is used along with the coffee enemas in the Gerson Therapy. Other modalities have been added to the Gerson Therapy; one most recently added is the use of ozone.

In the past many people have successfully treated themselves by studying and following the instructions in Dr. Gerson's popular book, *The Gerson Therapy 50 Case Histories.*

Today they can receive personal treatment at the CHIPSA Medical Center, eight miles from the Tijuana border, under the care and direction of Charlotte Gerson Strauss, Dr. Gerson's daughter, and her staff of professionally trained doctors and nurses.

The recommended stay at the Gerson Center is three weeks. Approximate cost is $4,000 a week.

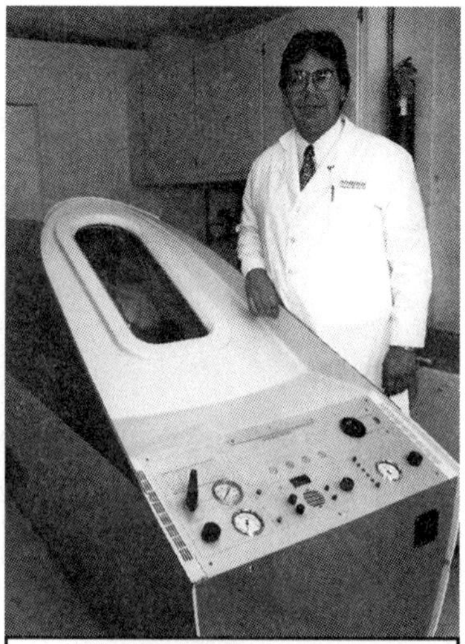

Hyberbaric Oxygen Chamber

- Specialty: melanoma, brain, liver, lupus, diabetes

Charlotte Gerson Strauss

Charlotte Gerson Strauss was born and had her schooling in Germany. She left in 1933 and continued school in Austria, France, and England, and attended Smith College after coming to New York. She helped translate her father's books and writings into English. She sometimes managed Dr. Gerson's clinics, attended his lectures, supervised nursing, and joined him in making rounds and in discussing cases. As president of the Gerson Institute, she lectures widely and teaches physicians who operate the CHIPSA Hospital in Tijuana.

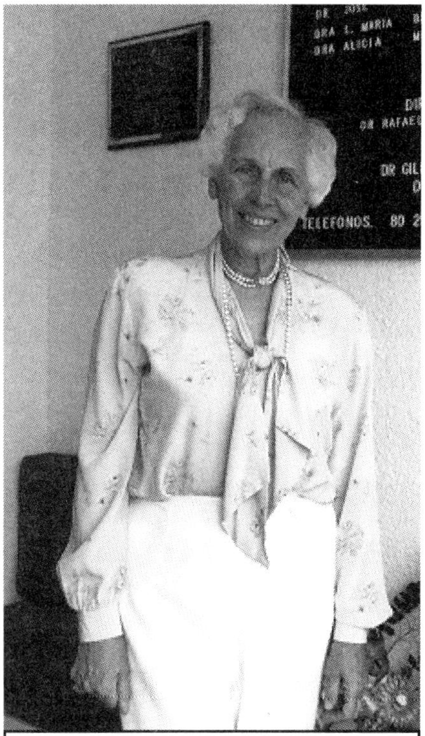

Charlotte Gerson Strauss

Tribute from Dr. Albert Schweitzer

Dr. Max Gerson is famous for his revolutionary healing therapy for cancer and other diseases. Dr. Albert Schweitzer called Dr. Gerson "one of medicine's most eminent geniuses."

Dr. Gerson saved Dr. Schweitzer's wife from hopeless lung tuberculosis in 1931 and healed their daughter of a rare, "incurable" erupting skin condition that defied diagnosis. Dr. Schweitzer himself came to Dr. Gerson at age 75 depressed and weary with advanced diabetes. In a few weeks Dr. Schweitzer was completely off his heavy insulin dosage, healed very well and had new energy and optimism. He returned to Africa where he won the Nobel Prize and worked past age 90.

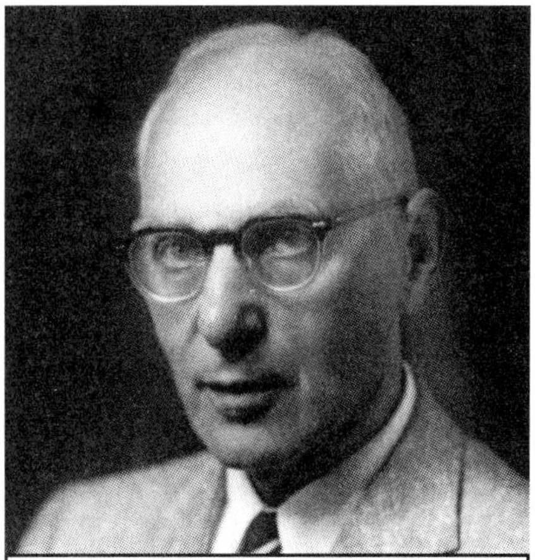

Dr. Max Gerson

Manner Clinic

Manner Clinic, Apartado 3437 Tijuana, B.C. Mexico
For mailing: P.O. Box 4290 San Ysidro, CA 92073
(800) 433-4962, (305) 454-8969
Reservations: 011-52-66-80-4222

"If you have a three-quarter inch cancerous tumor on your leg, the procedure is to cut off that leg. Well, we don't do that in metabolic therapy. Doesn't it make sense that if the body can reject a heart the size of your fist, that it can reject a three-quarter inch tumor?"
Dr. Harold Manner (NHF Convention, 1980, San Diego)

The Manner Clinic was named after Harold Manner, formerly the head of the biochemistry department of Loyola University in Chicago, Illinois. Although not a medical doctor, he taught doctors how to pass their final examinations and has written several biochemistry textbooks.

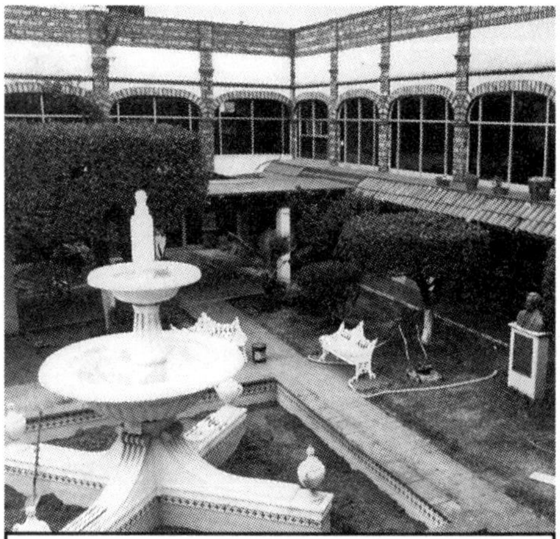

Manner Clinic

It was while working at Loyola University that Dr. Manner became interested in Laetrile. At the university he performed all the same tests on ice using Laetrile, vitamin A and enzymes just as Sloan Kettering and the National Cancer Institute had done. When he used mice that were tumor-induced, he got the same, unremarkable results as did all the other institutes. But he was still curious and did all the tests again on mice that automatically develop mammary tumors, and the results were significant: 75 percent regression. He then tested Laetrile, vitamin A and the enzymes separately and discovered that the enzymes were the most important of the three. He discovered the reason they worked so well was because the cancer had a protein shell around the tumors that could be broken down with the use of enzymes. "It is then that the Laetrile can do its work." The Laetrile is not a free cyanide until it reaches the cancer which has an enzyme called beta glucosidase and that activates the Laetrile to release the cyanide that starts to kill the cancer. The good cells are protected from the cyanide by rhodanese.

Dr. Manner knew that there was a great difference between men and mice and he asked some physician friends if they would incorporate these vitamins and enzymes into their patients' programs. They did, and had remarkable results. He then asked some metabolic physicians from all over the United States to join him. Most of these doctors were chiropractors as many M.D.'s did not want to get involved with the Laetrile controversy. Some of the doctors who joined him thought that metabolic treatment was anyone who prescribed vitamins to their patients—so then Dr. Manner went around every weekend, all over the United States, teaching doctors how to use the Manner therapy.

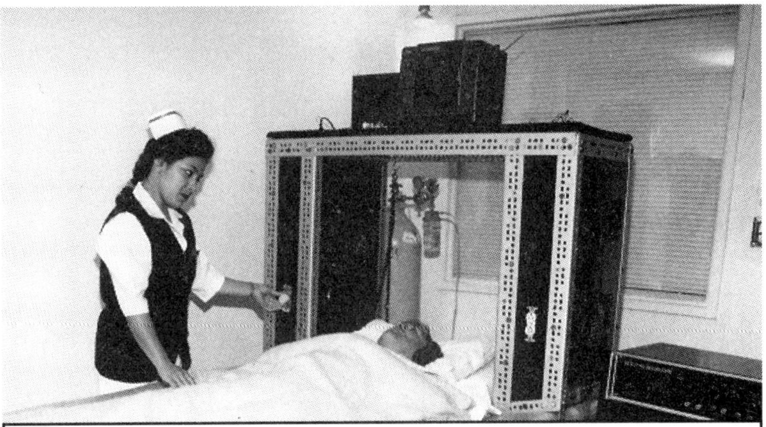

Patient Treatment

Every patient in every Manner Metabolic Clinic is put on a central computer which is located in Chicago. Available from this computer are the protocols for other degenerative diseases, including rheumatoid arthritis, multiple sclerosis and osteoarthritis.

The results are available to all the Manner clinics to aid the doctors in giving their patients the best of care. There are over 100 Manner Metabolic Clinics in the United States, Canada, Africa, Scotland and Japan. The Manner Clinic in Tijuana, Mexico, includes a hospital where he personally supervises every patient. At the Tijuana clinic the Manner therapy uses what is called the "Manner Cocktail." It is composed of 5 percent dextrose; 25,000 milligrams injectable vitamin C; 9 grams of Laetrile; and 10 cc of 99.9 injectable DMSO. This is all given in an I.V. drip.

Lodging is available adjoin-ing the Manner Complex and the Clinic's cafeteria pro-vides for the special required diet. The recommended stay at the Manner Clinic is three weeks. The cost is approx-imately $6,000 to $12,000.

- Specialty: brain, breast, arthritis, M.S

Harold Manner, Ph.D.

Dr. Manner received his Ph.D. from Northwestern University, Evanston, IL. in 1952.

His professional positions have been: visiting assistant professor of Biology, Ken-yon College, Gambier, Ohio, 1952-53; Associate professor of Biology, Utica College of Syracuse University 1953-62; Professor of Biology and Chairman of Division of Science and Mathematics, Utica College of Syracuse University, Utica, NY 1963-69; Professor of Biology and Chairman of the Biology Department, St. Louis University, St. Louis MO., 1969-72 and former Professor of Biology of the Biology Department, Loyola University, Chicago, IL.

Dr. Manner has biographical listings in "American Men of Science" and Who's Who in America". His numerous publications include textbooks on Anatomy and Physiology, Vertebrate Embryology and General Biology.

Some of his publications dealing with cancer are: The Non-toxicity of Amygdalin to Laboratory mice. Trans. IL. Acad. Sci.1977; The Effect of Amygdalin (Laetrile) on Pluripotential Fibroblast cells. Trans. IL. Acad. Sci. 1977; Enzymatic Analysis of Normal and Malignant Tissues. Trans. IL. Acad. Sci. 1978; Non-toxicity of Amygdalin to Mouse Fetuses. Trans. IL. Acad. Sci. 1978; End Products of Amygdalin Metabolism, Trans. IL. Acad. Sci. 1978. He co-authored The Death of Cancer, has 3 cassette tapes on Cancer, Arthritis and MS Therapy.

Dr. Manner is the President of the Metabolic Research Foundation, Glenview, IL. Currently, there are 168 Manner Clinics United States, Canada, Africa, Hawaii, Scotland and Japan. The latest in Tijuana is where he personally supervises every patient.

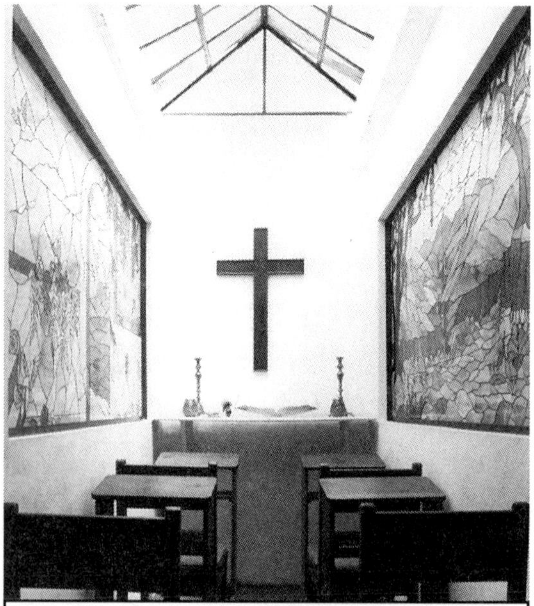

Chapel

Hospital Santa Monica
Donsbach Metabolic Therapy

Donsbach Metabolic Therapy
Rosarito Beach, Baja, Mexico
For mailing: 870 Canarios Court
Chula Vista, CA 91910
Mobile phone to clinic: (619) 428-1146
(800) 359-6457

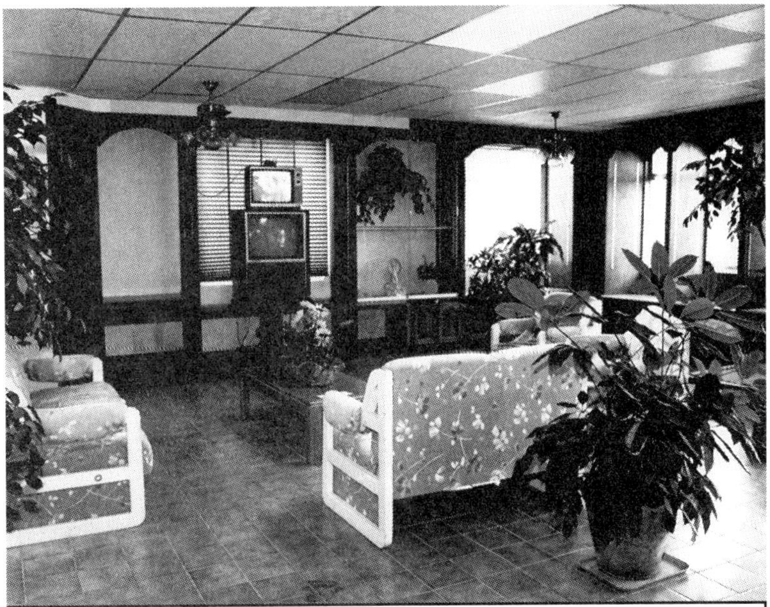

Hospital Santa Monica—Recreation Area

Dr. Kurt W. Donsbach had a dream to inform all people of their right to be self-educated regarding their own health.

Out of the not-so-available medical books and into the hands of anyone came countless publications—*Dr. Donsbach Tells You What You Always Wanted to Know About*—which have sold over eight million copies.

Recognizing the need for changes in nutritional standards and teachers to teach them, Dr. Donsbach established the Donsbach University School of Nutrition in Huntington Beach, California. The college's off-campus program afforded students from all over the world to obtain Dr. Donsbach's special nutritional degree, special because to become accredited meant his students had to learn more than any other student of nutrition. They had to have the credits required of the old school of nutrition plus all his new standardized classes on nutrition.

Dr. Donsbach had written books and taught teachers the new way to health and he wanted to create more than just a hospital. He wanted not only to create a place to get well, but a place to be revisited on a timely basis so that people could remain well. For this reason Hospital Santa Monica, a fully staffed hospital, offers also a lifetime, once a year, rejuvenation program at a minimal cost.

What does the Donsbach Hospital and Rejuvenation Program consist of? In general four approaches are used: intravenous infusion, intramuscular injections, nutritional support and physiotherapy.

The intravenous infusions may contain any number of substances chosen from a master list according to the needs of the patient. Some substances used regularly are vitamins, minerals, amino acids and hydrogen peroxide. Although growth hormone therapy is not used as a main part of the treatment, it is used as an adjunct to assist in the restoration of normal function in the brain, lungs, heart, kidneys, spleen, thymus, adrenals, thyroid and pituitary glands.

For cancer patients, Laetrile, special thymus extract, tumorex, hydrazine sulfate, ozone and/or GH3 may be used.

Intramuscular injections contain smaller amounts of the same ingredients contain-ed in the I.V., with exception of amino acids. This method is used as an alternative to the I.V.

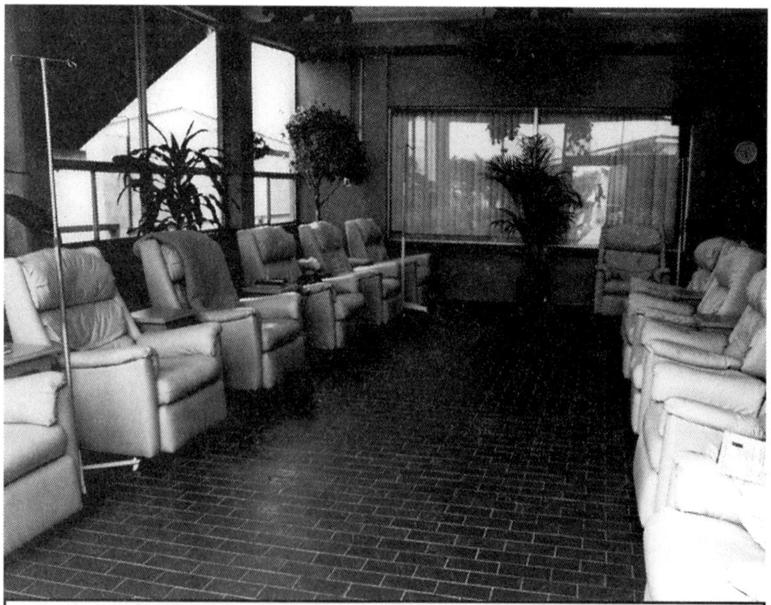

Chelation and Nutritional I.V. Room

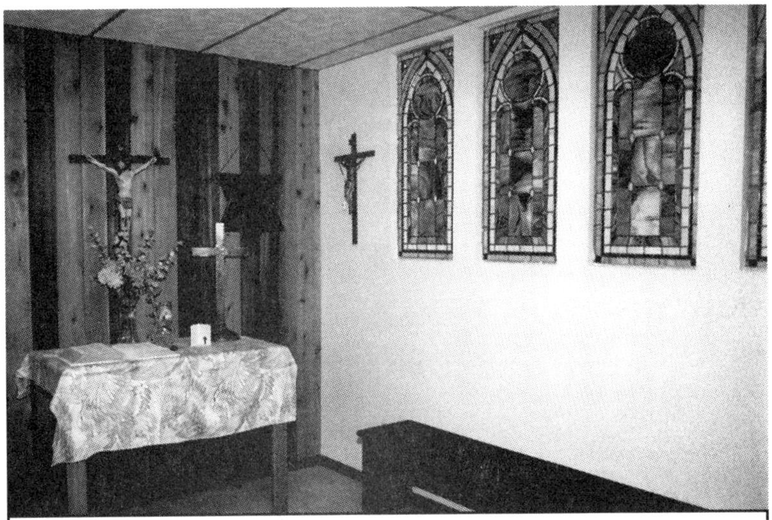

Chapel

Nutritional support consists of dietary supplementation according to the individual patient's needs. The food served at Hospital Santa Monica is high in fiber and low in sugar. Correct food combining is encouraged for better digestion and assimilation. Hydrochloric acid and digestive enzyme supplements are provided at each meal. Nutritional counseling regarding the detriments of salt and sugar is also part of the "taking responsibility for your diet" program. Physiotherapy and hydro-therapy consist of massage, sauna baths, whirlpool baths, swimming, exercise and colonics. Chiropractic and dental services are also available through Hospital Santa Monica.

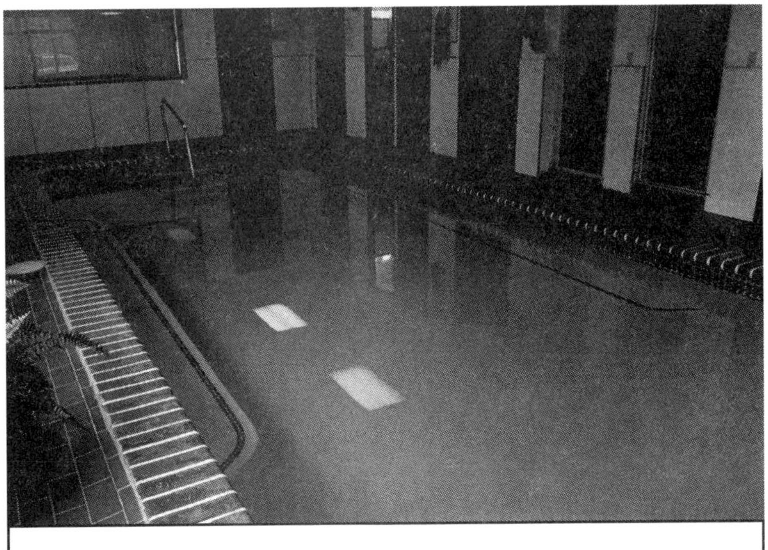

Pool

The recommended stay is three weeks. Hospital Santa Monica also provides an out-patient program. Patients take home any equipment issued to them during the program that may be deemed necessary for their recovery. A three week stay may cost from $8,000 to $12,000. Visa and Mastercard are accepted.

- Specialty: degenerative diseases, rejuvenation

Kurt Donsbach, Ph.D.

Kurt Donsbach, Ph.D. began his career in the healing arts as a physician specializing in the treatment of arthritis and rheumatoid disorders. Later, he accepted a position with the famous Dr. Royal Lee of the Lee Foundation for Nutritional Research where he assisted in the development of wholistic treatments for the treatment of arthritis without pain killers.

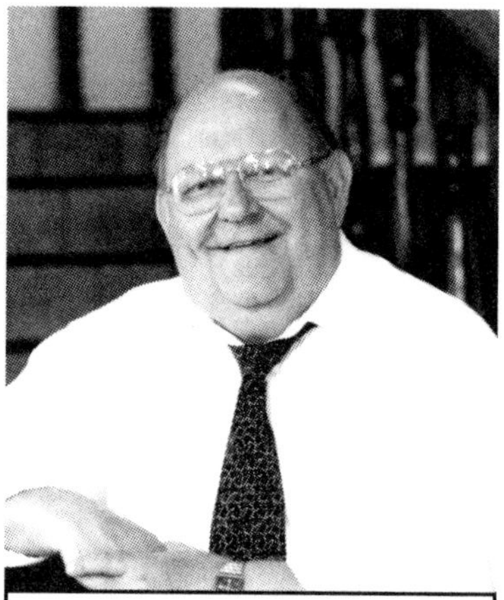

Dr. Kurt Donsbach

Currently, he is President of Donsbach University, School of Nutrition, with overseas campuses in Israel, Japan, Canada, South Africa, and West Germany. He serves as Chairman of the Board of Governors of the National Health Federation and President of the International Institute of Natural Health Sciences. He has appeared on numerous radio and television shows and currently has his own radio show called *Let's Talk Health* in Southern California, on KPEZ-AM and 10:00 a.m.

In addition to his best seller book, *Supernutrition*, Dr. Donsbach has authored over 40 publications on the subject of nutrition. His *Dr. Donsbach Tells You What You Always Wanted To Know About* series has sold over 8 million copies.

Dr. Donsbach is currently Director of the Biogenesis Institute, a wholistic care facility located in Rosarito Beach, Baja, California.

St. Jude's International
Keller Metabolic Therapy

St. Jude's International—Keller Metabolic Therapy
911 Television (Clinic Juarez) Centro-Medical-Tijuana
c/o Ron Keller P.O. Box 125 Westcliff, CO 81252
(303) 783-2703
011-52-66-847333 (10 a.m. - 2 p.m.)
(706) 681-3026 (evenings)

In 1968 Jimmy Keller was diagnosed as having a malignant melanoma of the left ear.

He was told since radiation and chemotherapy were not effective treatments, he would have to have his ear, part of his jaw and the muscle from the left side of his neck removed. Two months after his operation, a knot on his neck returned and soon more knots under his arms and in his chest. He felt betrayed since this time he had to have the radiation which was supposed to be ineffective the first time.

Jimmy felt prayer played an important role in his recovery. His mother and father had been making novenas to Saint Jude and soon after his mother received an anonymous letter telling of an herbal treatment in Dallas, Texas. This therapy was soon to be moved to Tijuana, Mexico. To please his mother and father, Jimmy went to Dallas for treatment. While there he learned of other alternative treatments like the Gerson and Laetrile therapies and he started combining them with his herbal treatment.

Because of his failure with orthodox therapy and his success with alternative therapies, Jimmy wanted to inform other people who had cancer. He first recommended that they go to the alternative cancer clinics in Tijuana. Some of them did go to Tijuana, but when they returned home there wasn't anyone to help them with their injections. Doctors and nurses were afraid of losing their licenses and would not get involved. Jimmy decided that he could and would give the injections himself. "My home in Baton Rouge became a 'Mecca' for people with cancer. I operated out of my home for seven years, often seeing more than 100 patients a week." Jimmy learned of chelation therapy from Dr. Ray Evers and it was soon included in treatments as well as enzymes and herbs.

Jimmy felt that he was getting as well as, if not at least equally good, results with his protocol as were the treatments given in Tijuana. He wanted people to know of his success and started lecturing all over the state.

Six years ago Jimmy's melanoma returned. By using amino acid formulas he recovered his health. He felt that these amino acid formulas were the most effective modality that he had used so far and he began integrating them into his cancer patients' programs.

Jimmy still could not find licensed doctors and nurses who could help and was soon forced to leave his state and to join other physicians in Tijuana, Mexico.

Other modalities that the clinic uses include radionics to balance the body's energy fields. There is an emphasis on maintaining, in the colon, a clean environment and good bacteria. Positive mind therapy with the use of daily repetitive affirmations is also used.

Patients are tested daily with kinesiology to see which modality will be effective for them.

Although a relatively new clinic in Tijuana, the Keller Metabolic Therapy has been reported to be successful as well as fast—that is, tumors are said to be reduced in size as much as one cm every three days.

Patients come to St. Jude's Clinic located in the Tijuana Medical Center on an out-patient basis. They are advised to stay in Tijuana for at least two weeks. The total cost of the Keller treatments is about $3,200.)

More Mexico & Tijuana Clinics

- Cydel Medical Center
  P.O. Box 434290
  San Ysidro, CA 92143
  011-52-66-804-422
  800-248-8431
- Stella Maris Clinic
  Filberto Alvarzi, MD
  P.O. Box 435123
  San Ysidro, CA 92143
  011-52-66-343444
  800-662-1319
- Bio-energetic Clinic
  Gerald Hall, DC
  10904 Lakewood Ave.
  El Paso, Tx 79935
  9155980601
- Centre Nueve Vida
  San Chachona, M.D.
  190 E. Calle Premivera, #235
  San Ysidro, CA 90273
  011-53-66-863-161/30071
  619-6622730
- Institure of Chronic Diseases
  Gustao Andrado, M.D.
  416 W. San Ysidro, Bldg.#677
  San Ysidro, CA 90273
  011-52-66-341026
- International Medical Center
  F. Soto M.D.
  R. James M.D.
  1420 Geronimo Dr., #D-2
  El Paso, Tx 79925
- St. Luke International Hospital
  416 W. San Ysidro Blvd. #L-214
  San Ysidro CA, 92143
  800-231-1088
- Charles Rogers, M.D.
  507 E. Elizabeth Street
  Brownsville, TX 78520
  210-541-7182
- Jaime Narvaez
  P.O. Box 10235
  El Paso, Tx 79993
  800-862-8881
  011-52-16-135931

PART III

"Chew your liquids and drink your foods."
Gandhi

Dr. Javier Morales, D.D.S.

Multualismo 1217 (corner of 6th St.)
Tijuana, B.C. Mexico
001-52-66-883242
Fax: 001-52-66-3248

"We will not put anything in your mouth that will harm your body." This is the basis of our practice.

Dr. Javier Morales, D.D.S., is probably the most famous alternative dentist in Tijuana, Mexico. Working with the alternative physicians for many years, he has gained respect from patients and their doctors for his specialized dentistry.

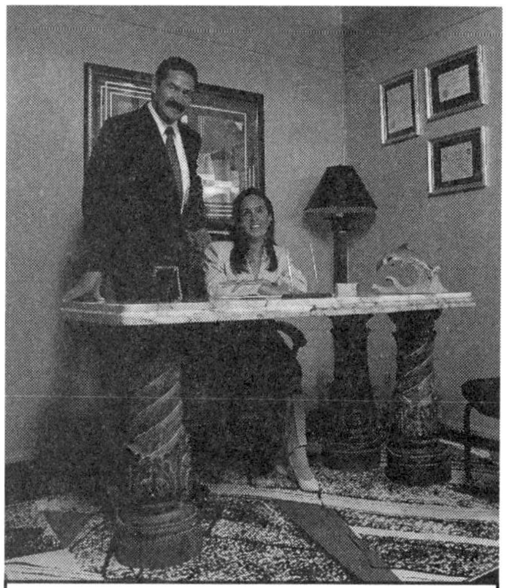

Dr. Javier Morales, D.D.S.

The removal of silver mercury fillings has become a major part of alternative medicine in the treatment of cancer and other degenerative diseases. The alternative physician and the alternative dentist work side by side to reassure their patients' immune systems can achieve maximum performance.

Dr. Morales says, "Amalgam fillings, root canals, porcelain crowns and fixed bridges are bad news. Under each porcelain crown or bridge is a metal base made of nickel alloy. Exposure to nickel alloy can cause cancer of the lungs, nasal passages and larynx. Root canals produce bacteria that can become toxic poisons in the body, triggering heart disease, arthritis and osteitis of the jaw."

"Amalgam fillings have been used for 150 years. Amalgam is 50 percent mercury, a deadly poison. Mercury poison migrates in your body for up to five years. Mercury vapor poison settles in brain tissue. Decay is common under metal fillings. Body and mouth bacteria mix with mercury to form methyl mercury, a substance 100 times more toxic."

"Saliva acts as an electrolyte when it mixes with amalgam fillings, to create a measurable electric current of 900 millivolts. This current overpowers the body's normal 450 millivolts, interferes with energy flow to the brain and is suspect as a catalyst in many illnesses. With this, many common substances, such as caffeine, inhibit your body's cleansing process."

"Mercury poison is also linked to birth defects."

Dr. Javier Morales is a research pioneer in modern holistic dentistry. He specializes in successful removal of amalgam fillings, nickel crowns, root canal cavitations, and overcoming mercury poisoning.

While at the Morales clinic, special safety procedures are used to protect the dental patient: An electrical readout of each filling is done before removal. Rubber dam, oxygen

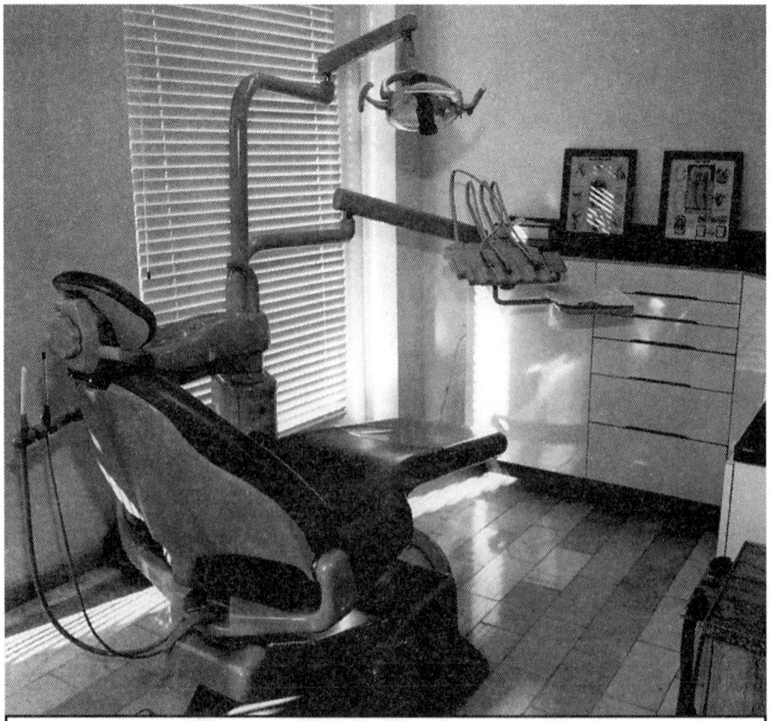

Dental Room

nose mask and high-powered vacuums are used. Ceramic reinforced resin is used to help make filled teeth solid and leave no room for decay under the filling. Intravenous vitamin C is also available.

Sterilization procedures include: ultrasonic machine cleaning; detergent soaking and washing; 10 hour chemical solution soak; individualized sterilization bag for each patient; 45 minute quemiclave per bag (stronger than autoclave); disposable or personalized hand piece; ion generator in area; and dental chairs are sterilized after each patient.

A shuttle bus is made available to and from a California motel for patients who want to make a long appointment to minimize travel. Most United States insurance coverage is accepted.

Additional Dental Clinic

The Castillo Clinic
Dr. Silva Palacios Roji

PART IV

"The nomenclature of diseases from their remote cause is the most offensive and injurious part of the rubbish of our science. The physician who can cure one disease by a knowledge of its principles may by the same means cure all of the diseases of the human body; for their causes are the same." —Dr. Benjamin Rush

Metabolic Cancer Therapy

METABOLIC THERAPY

According to the dictionary, "metabolic" means pertaining to metabolism. It says that metabolism is the sum of all physical and chemical changes that take place in an organism. Therefore, to treat a person metabolically is to pay particular attention to the chemical balances that go on in the body and to make changes when indicated. Now, to start to do this there must first be a set of standards that describe what normal is for the human body. The metabolic physician often uses two sets of standards: the one set by modern medicine and a metabolic standard like the Manner Normal Blood Profile. (See page 51—Manner Normal Blood Profile chart.)

If urine and blood tests are taken and an individual is determined not to have a chemical imbalance, then the metabolic physician will proceed to make the proper changes to bring the body back into balance (such as the acid/alkaline of the small intestine or of the stomach or colon). If a person is deficient in particular vitamins or minerals, then those are supplemented.

Few or many modalities may be used to achieve the correct balance. Some of the most common modalities are fresh and raw organically grown fruits and vegetables and their juices, vaccines, and cellular therapy. By balancing the body's chemistry, the immune system is given a chance to function properly and the body will make an effort to heal itself. A common method of administration in metabolic therapy is an I.V. drip.

DETOXIFICATION

If the body is toxic and this toxicity is making the chemical imbalance, then steps are taken to detoxify the person. This may be done with herbal laxatives, coffee enemas and/or colonics.

CANCER SYMPTOM

The parasite (the wound, infection, or tumor) is also treated, but the main focus in metabolic therapy is on the host (the body). The reason being, which has been observed clinically, that when all is done that can be done for the host, then the parasite (the tumor), just as it appeared from within, can disappear the same way.

Periodic testing is then done to see if the assigned program is working for an individual and changes are made accordingly.

TESTS

Regular blood and urine tests are given by the medical metabolic doctor, but the methods of diagnosing are much more complex and usually include a few more tests. These additional tests may include kinesiology, hair analysis, darkfield or live blood test. Tests are given throughout therapy, and sometimes daily, to determine efficacy of modalities, and changes are made accordingly. These cancer monitoring tests are sometimes referred to as "cancer monitors."

Cancer and precancer tests, like the Navarro or Neunhoeffer Tests, are sometimes given. Some of these tests can detect the probability of cancer, from and up to, eight years before the appearance of a tumor. It is said that they can determine the strength of the immune system. If the immune tests show a deficiency, immune-enhancing vitamins like A or C, or glandulars like thymus, or immune-enhancing vaccines like autogenous or BCG, may be added to the metabolic program.

For more about test information see PART IX.

BLOOD TESTS

Laboratory norms for blood profiles represent an average of the population. If the population becomes sicker, the ranges become greater. For this reason the norms accompanying the blood tests do not represent ideal conditions from a metabolic therapy viewpoint. It is suggested that the following ranges be substituted:

MANNER NORMAL BLOOD PROFILE

Manner Normal Blood Profile

Terms	Values	Terms	Values
Calcium	9.7-10.1	Potassium "serum"	4.0-4.3
Phosophorus	3.1-3.5	Chloride "serum"	100-104
Glucose	85-100	Creatinine "serum"	0.7-1.0
Bun	13-17	Iron "serum"	95-100
Uric Acid	4.5-5.5	Bun/creatinine ratio	14.5-15.5
Cholesterol	185-215	Triglycerides9	5-105
Total protein	7.2-7.5	WBC	5000-6000
Albumen	4.0-4.4	RBC	4.5-5.0 million
Bilirubin	0.5-0.7	Hemoglobin	14.5-15.0 GM%
Alkaline phosphatase	10-50	Hematocrit	40-50%
Acid phosphatase	0-2	Eosinophils	0-2%
LDH	125-135	Basophils	0-2%
SGOT	18-22	Monocytes	4-6%
Total globulin	2.8-3.5	Lymphocytes	34-45%
A/G ratio	2.5-3.5	Segs	45-55%
Sodium "serum"	140-143		

CANCER PROBABILITY TEST

Navarro Table of Values

(from Navarro Cancer Probability Test)

Index	Int. Units	New Interpretation
0	0	Negative
1-3	1-49	Doubtful
4	50-400	Faintly positive
5	401-1000	Moderately positive
6	1001-3000	Definitely positive
7	3001-5000	Heavily positive
8	5001-10,000	Very heavily positive
9	10,000 and over	Excessively positive

For more about test information see Part IX.

EXTERNAL DETOXIFICATION

Patients are counseled regarding their external environment and made aware of possible existing carcinogens. They may be told to stop using hair dyes or deodorants and toothpaste that contain aluminum by-products. Air and water purifiers may be recommended. The use of natural fabrics like cotton will be encouraged, or the removal of silver/mercury fillings and their replacement with a lesser or non-toxic substance: All of this to help the immune system to function at a higher level.

PHYSICAL THERAPY

Our lymphatic system cannot function without our movement. For this reason any amount of exercise or movement is recommended and almost always a part of treatment. The physical well-being and comfort of the patient is very important in metabolic therapy. Some metabolic clinics include hydrotherapy, saunas, massage, floatation tanks, light therapy and/or herbal baths.

MIND AND SPIRIT

Mind and spirit therapy may also be a part of the metabolic patient's program. This may include meditation, prayer, emotional or psychological counseling. Imaging may also be recommended.

METABOLIC THERAPY FROM A LECTURE BY DR. ERNESTO CONTRERAS TREATMENT AND MANAGEMENT OF CANCER IN THE UNITED STATES

Theories About Cancer Development From a lecture by Dr. Ernest Contreras

From a lecture by Dr Ernesto Contreras

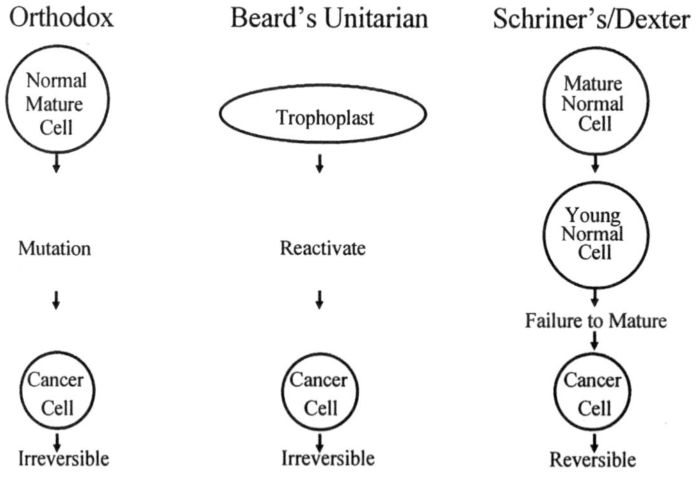

All efforts in orthodox therapy is to kill the parasite and nothing is done to help the Host. They have been treating cancer like this for 100 years.

CONTRERAS LECTURE ABOUT CANCER DEVELOPMENT

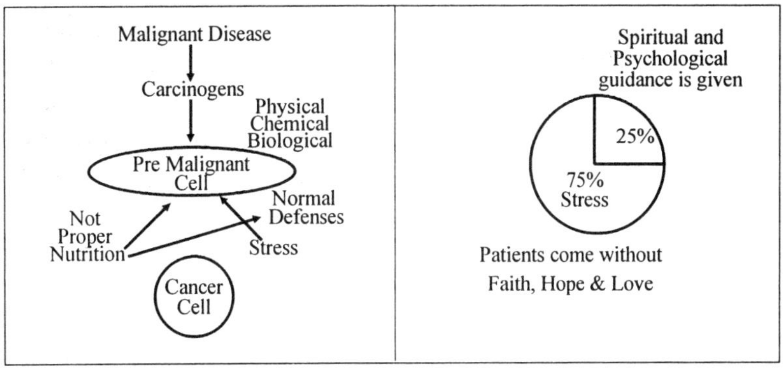

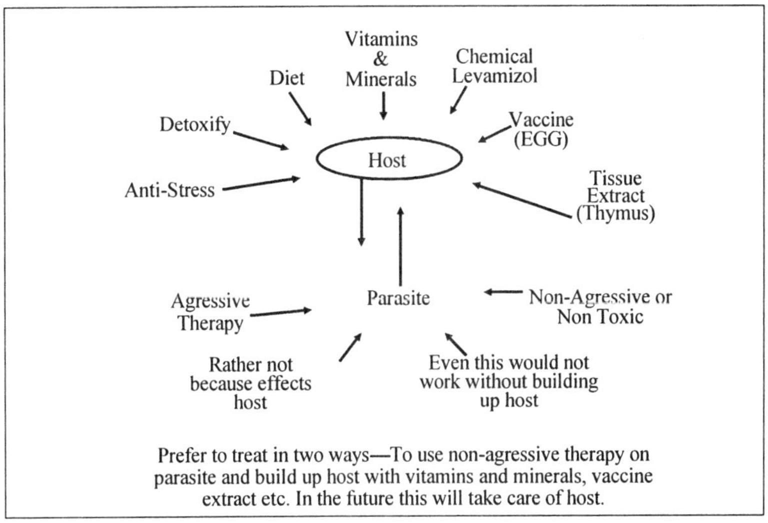

CANCER IN THE UNITED STATES:

Symptoms of Cancer: Usually a tumor
Diagnostic Tests: Palpation, X-ray, biopsy, surgery
Treatment: Chemotherapy, radiation, surgery, hormones.

CANCER IN TIJUANA:

Symptoms: Usually a tumor
Diagnostic Tests: Same as for precancer plus palpation and X-ray
Treatment: Same as for precancer

PRECANCER OR PROBABILITY OF CANCER IN TIJUANA, MEXICO (ALSO AVAILABLE IN U.S.):

Symptoms of Cancer: Usually no physical or visible signs. Sometimes can be seen in iris (Iridology tests)
Diagnostic Tests: Blood (AMID, CEA) and urine (Navarro) (protein) (Neunhoffer) (Norton)
Accompanying Tests: (May be) hair analysis, SMAC 24, Darkfield, HCG
Treatment: External and internal detoxification, diet, vitamins and minerals, enzymes, immunology, stress reduction.

CANCER'S PROTEIN SHELL

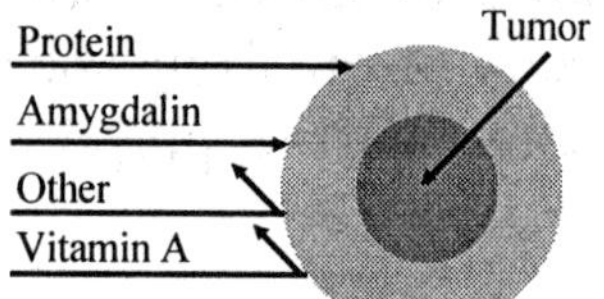

A representation of a Tumor Cell with the surrounding Protein Coat

The Protein Coat surrounding the tumor mass may act as a barrier for most tumoricidal agents rendering them ineffective on the tumor

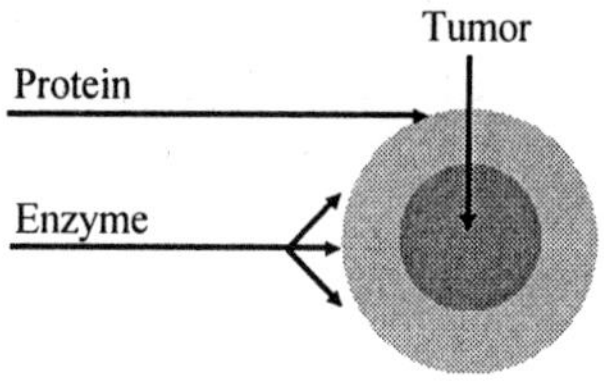

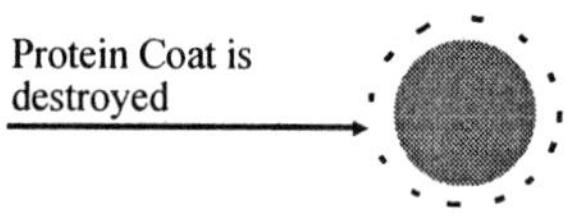

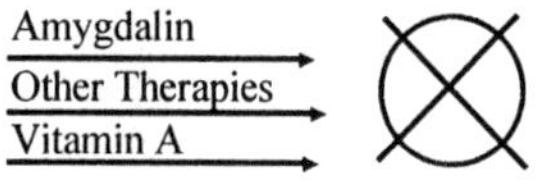

The effects of the enzyme complex on the Protein Coat allows various therapies to attack the tumor

Once the Protein Coat, which surrounds the malignancy is destroyed, amygdalin and vitamin A are able to attack the tumor.

Cancers 'Protected' By Cocoons

BOSTON (AP) — Many types of cancer may spread - protected by the body's natural disease defenses - because they exist within cocoons of gel made by the tumors themselves.

In a three-year study on animals released Sunday, researchers identified several of the substances secreted by the tumors and described how the protective environments are fashioned.

The researchers found the substances in two kinds of cancer in guinea pigs and cautioned they are not certain the phenomenon works exactly the same way in human beings.

But they said their study may lead to new ways of treating cancer in humans.

The work, conducted at Massachusetts General Hospital, was published in the Journal of the National Cancer Institute.

Dr. Harold Dvorak, chief of the hospital's immunopathology unit, said his research team found that tumors live inside cocoons made of a substance called fibrin gel.

Normally, the body's immune system finds proteins called antigens on the surface of the tumor cells and treats them as foreign invaders. However, inside the cocoons, the tumors are safe from detection.

The blood contains two proteins - fibrinogen, which helps blood clot, and plasminogen, which dissolves clots.

Dvorak said the tumor secretes an agent that causes blood vessels to lead. Then a substance secreted by the tumor converts the fibrinogen to fibrin gel.

"If the tumor only laid down the gel around it, it would trap itself and be unable to grow," Dvorak said. "So the tumor also produces material to convert the plasminogen into a very active enzyme which dissolves fibrin. The result is that as more gel collects on the outer fringe of the cocoon, fibrin closest to the tumor itself is eliminated, thus allowing the tumor to expand."

In this way, the doctor said, the tumor turns the body's own mechanisms to the advantage of the disease.

"I think the latest studies may ultimately open the door to a whole new approach to tumor treatment," Dvorak said.

—Reprinted from The Register, Santa Ana, CA, Aug. 6, 1979

LIVE CELL THERAPY

In 1930 with the discovery of Rh factors in blood, the first blood banks were established. Prior to that time, attempted transfusions were denounced as some kind of witch-doctoring.

Fortunately sense overcame these narrow views and soon accepted even bone marrow transplantation as another way to save lives.

Today we accept the crisis transplantation of kidneys, veins, livers and even hearts. Logic tells us, though, that prevention is better than crisis organ transplants and that cellular implantation may provide an important avenue in that direction.

Cellular implantation, better known as growth hormone therapy, is the preparation of cells taken from specific organs of an unborn animal fetus for the purpose of injection into a human recipient.

The cells are taken from animals that have been bred and maintained specifically for that purpose.

When the cells are injected into the human recipient, they travel to the similar organ from which they were taken, to revitalize and stimulate that organ's function. Dr. Schmid and H. Lettre at the Heidelberg University conclusively demonstrated, by radio tagging and tracing specific organ cells from a fetal donor, that the host's bloodstream transported the vast majority of the cells to the counterpart organ of the host.

The underlying of live cells therapy is equivalent to infusing an old tree with a hundred-thousand-fold young buds. These buds will graft onto the limbs and produce roots and shoots that will enable that tree to flourish and luxuriate.

In 1931, Professor Paul Niehans, a Swiss surgeon, became interested in endocrinology and studied the work of his colleagues experimenting with the implantation of animal glands into patients whose organs were not functioning properly. Dr. Niehans' research led to the conclusions that, while the functions of all corresponding mammalian organs (congeneric organs) are almost identical, there are certain subtle differentiations of cell content that make them, most often, not compatible or transferable between species. This wasn't true, he determined, for the cells of organs still developing in the fetal stage.

Fetal cells are not recognized by the body as being foreign. They remain undetected and so, to a certain extent, can become new building blocks to restore specific worn or ailing organs.

Dr. Niehans observed that after the injection of cells from specific organs, the function of the corresponding human organ almost invariably improves. This has been validated by scientifically-controlled laboratory and clinical experiments. In the 40 years following his first successful experiments, Professor Niehans applied his discoveries in cellular therapy over 50,000 times.

Symptoms indicative of cell therapy are subnormal functioning of gland, premature aging, chronic degenerative disease, susceptibility to infection and disease, maldevelopment in infancy such as Down's Syndrome, birth injuries, encephalitis, and CP.

BIO-ELECTRIC MEDICINE

Every human function and thought is transmitted by the conduction of electrical signals. Life could not exist at all without a constant flow of ions across the membrane of the cell's wall. At the cellular level, electrical changes take place between the potassium in the cell and the sodium outside the cell.

Consider the cells, tissues, organs, the interstitial fluid, blood vessels, lymphatic channels and excretory canals within the body as functioning the same way as insulated electrical cables, blood plasma conducting currents effectively inside the relatively insulated vessel walls to join the conducting interstitial tissue fluid over the blood capillaries.

The Bio-Electric Activator is used to change the electrical currents of the body. By changing these currents, the electrical fields are also changed throughout the body, the current flowing, preferably in conducting pathways including ionic and electro-osmatic transports and over both short and long distances, produces a diverse biological effect.

The idea is that the electricity can stimulate bodily defenses, alert repair mechanisms and control the growth and function of cells. Bio-electric is not a new concept to medicine. Dr. Samuel C. West has been teaching that body cells are electrical for over 12 years.

His research has proven how and why bio-electric cell activation works. First pioneered in Sweden by Bjorn Nordenstrom and in North America by Dr. Gary Young, bio-electric medicine has been shown to be an effective treatment for cancer, multiple sclerosis and other degenerative diseases.

Over the past 14 years the research work conducted by Dr. Nordenstrom with lung and breast cancer has resulted in over 75 percent remissions.

CHELATION

The word chelation comes from a Greek word that means to claw.

Chelation Therapy is done with an IV drip with EDTA. There are other ingredients that can basically accomplish the same thing, EDTA takes the plaque or fatty deposits from the body as well as some mineral deposits. After therapy, a person is usually injected with beneficial minerals or they are added in the IV drip near the end of the therapy. The therapy lasts for 3 to 4 hours. Severity of accumulated minerals, such as lead, mercury, aluminum or other circulatory impairments will determine the number of chelation therapies given. The number may be anywhere from 6 to 30.

There is some evidence that chelation therapy has enabled some people to by-pass their by-pass operations. It has been beneficial in the treatment of cancer patients by improving circulation and enabling metabolic therapy to work faster.

Chelation was first used on lead poisoned patients. It was discovered that these patients did not acquire the usual heart problems as did most of the general population.

Vitamins B and C are sometimes added to the IV drip.

This therapy is available in the United States as well.

COLONICS AND COLEMAS

There are various ways of cleansing the colon. Some work faster than others.

The colonic is a machine that puts water into the colon and at the same time takes water and waste out with the use of two small hoses.

The colema is used with a colema board and a five gallon bottle hung above. The person using this method is able to adjust the flow of water. The tube or hose in the rectum is very small and allows for the waste to bypass it. Sometime chaparrel tea or other ingredients are added to the water.

HOMEOPATHY

You have heard, "cures like cures", but what does that mean?

It was Samual Hahnermann who realized that illness was a curative process and developed this system of medicine we call "homeopathy".

Homeopathy comes from the Greek words homios, *like/similar*, and pathos, *sickness/suffering*. The homeopath administers highly diluted medically prescribed substances that are *like/similar* to a *sickness/suffering* in a patient, not to get rid of a disease but to stimulate the body's immune system to cure in the way it wants naturally and not the way of the physician.

Homeopathy views illness as a curative process that should not be interrupted, and that the symptoms should be stimulated not suppressed, such as is practiced in allopathy. The goal of homeopathy is to see a disease or illness through to the end. It is thought that to stop the curative process is to cause a greater illness in the future.

Advantages of homopathy are: no side effects, promotes natural healing and is relatively inexpensive.

HYPERTHERMIA

Hyperthermia is heat therapy.

It has been established that controlled elevation of temperature to the hyperthermia range of 108 to 113 degrees can selectively damage malignant tissue while leaving surrounding normal tissue unharmed.

Hyperthermia has also shown a synergistic effect when used with radio-therapy and some chemotherapies, and is able to reduce the amounts of radiotherapy and chemotherapy used.

Several different methods for delivery of heat to affected areas have been tried from hot water, hot covers, hot wax, and diverting blood through a special heater. The difficulty in the past has been to deliver heat evenly and in reaching as much of the tumor as possible and only the tumor.

Advances have been made by using a microwave hyperthermia machine consisting of an extendable arm linked to a control-box-like application that is placed on the patient directly over the tumor. Inside the applicator are antennas and by alternating the power supply to each one, the heat can be distributed directly and evenly to the tumor.

Hyperthermia has been particularly effective in reducing prostate swelling and rectal tumors.

LAETRILE

Derived from apricot kernels and is used in IV drips and/or given orally (usually 500mg.). The purpose of using Laetrile for cancer treatment is to break down tumor tissue. Laetrile is a free cyanide that is non-occurring until it reaches the tumor. The beta glucosidase in the tumor releases the cyanide in the Laetrile to fight the tumor. The good cells are protected by rhodanese. Mouse studies have shown Laetrile to be effective on automatically occurring breast tumors. Clinical studies have shown an effective reduction in breast cancer tumors.

OXYGEN THERAPIES

Since the loss of oxygen to nerves is the primary cause of long term injury, all types of oxygen therapies should be considered for use right after injury and for old injuries.

Although $H_2 0_2$ has its pros and cons regarding excessive use, it may provide oxygen to a new wound. ozone, Koch and Rodaquin (a cousin to Koch), are also oxygenators.

Because cancer cannot live in oxygen, the above mentioned therapies are being used in other countries to fight tumors.

Rodaquin is used in the United States in dermatology offices to help rid patients of scar tissue. In Tijuana, Mexico, it is used in some of the clinics to help M.S. patients regain more mobility. It works on the blockages in the spine.

ROCEPHINE

Injectable. Used in the States for spider bites. In Mexico it is used as an alternative to penicillin for the treatment in cancer. It is used to fight the almost always occurring infection associated with cancer. It doesn't have the usual side affects of other anti-bacterial agents.

THYMUS

Injectable and oral use. Used to build up the immune system. When tests (cancer markers) show a probability of future cancer (Neunhoeffer) thymus is administered.

SUGGESTED
DETOXIFICATION DIET

DIET FOR CANCER PATIENTS [1]		
	FOODS TO INCLUDE	FOODS TO AVOID
Beverages	Large amounts of fresh vegetable and fruit juices, especially carrot, greens, beet and apple. Herb teas, especially peppermint. Soya, sesame or nut milk.	White bread and white flour products such as macaroni, crackers and snack food.
Breads	Miller, rye, buckwheat, whole-wheat, bran, corn and soya. Corn tortillas. Only whole grains, freshly ground or spouted, free of additives. Avoid rancid flour. Use a flour mill.	Processed cereals, which are flaked, puffed, etc. No white rice.
Cereals	Miller, oatmeal, brown and wild rice, buckwheat groats, cornmeal, cracked wheat. Avoid rancid grains. Use a nut grinder.	Processed cereals, which are flaked, puffed, etc. No white rice.
Dairy	Unsweetened yogurt, cottage cheese, and raw certified milk, goat cheese, soya cheese.	Cheese, butter, and commercial milk.
Eggs	Poached or boiled fertile eggs used sparingly.	Fried and non-fertile eggs.
Fruits	All fresh fruits (organically grown): apples, apricots, bananas, cherries, berries, melon, papaya, pineapple, etc. Use citrus sparingly. Unsulphured dried fruit.	Sprayed, sweetened, frozen, and canned fruit. Sulphured dried fruit.
Meats	Fresh white-fleshed fish, lamb, buffalo, deer.	Shell-fish and all other meats. No fried, smoked, salted or processed meats. No nitrates, antibiotics or stilbesterol.
Oils	Most cold-pressed unsaturated oil, such as safflower, sesame, canola, olive, and avocado. Use sparingly. Avocado used whole may replace butter.	No cottonseed oil. No rancid or continuously heated oils. Shortening and margarine.
Nuts	Most fresh raw nuts, particularly almonds, cashew. Raw nut butters freshly made and refrigerated to avoid rancidity. Use sparingly.	Roasted and salted nuts, especially peanuts. Rancid nuts and nut butters.
Seasonings	Chives, garlic, parsley. Herbs: bay, basil, sage, thyme, savory, kelp, cayenne, cloves.	Salt
Seeds	Sunflower, pumpkin, sesame, chia and flax. Fruit kernels: apricot, apple, prune, plum, and peach.	Roasted and salted seeds.
Sprouts	Mung, alfalfa, lentil, soy, fenugreek, buckwheat, and wheat, which can be made into wheat grass juice.	Poisonous potato sprouts.
Sweets	Sorghum, raw honey, pure maple syrup, and carob used sparingly over cereal or in health deserts (with healthy ingredients).	White sugar and sugar substitutes. Chocolate. Commercial candies and pastries.
Vegetable	All raw or lightly steamed vegetables (organically grown). Homemade soups. Baked red potatoes.	Sprayed, frozen, and canned vegetables. French fried potatoes. Potato and corn chips.

Every individual is different and so are their dietary needs. This Suggested Detoxification Diet has been included in this publication because of the many requests for it and is not intended to be used for treatment of disease. It is recommended that you consult your metabolic physician for individualized and special diet programming.

[1]This diet can be more restricted according to the severity of the disease. Eliminate all dairy and meat during the first three weeks of detoxification.

PART V

"If I have told you earthly things, and ye believe not, how shall ye believe if I tell you of Heavenly things?"
—Jesus, St. John 3, Verse 12

Questions and Answers

23 Years of Questions

1. What is the difference in the treatment for cancer in Mexico and the United States?

In Mexico the cancer is treated, but also the person that has the cancer, the host. The parasite and the host. In America they treat the cancer. They take the tumor and they cut it and they radiate the person and they give them chemotherapy. No thought is given to the fact that this person is very, very sick and has developed this tumor, usually, because of a sick body. In Mexico, the whole body is treated. In some cases they do use surgery, and in some clinics they do use radiation and chemotherapy, but for the most part, first they use what we call holistic or metabolic therapy and do no harm to the body whenever possible.

2. What exactly is meant by metabolic treatment or metabolic therapy?

The dictionary refers to metabolic as pertaining to metabolism. Metabolism is the sum of all physical and chemical changes that take place in an organism. To treat a person metabolically is to pay particular attention to the chemical charges that go on in the body. A metabolic or nutritional doctor will give a blood test and a urine test to determine exactly what the chemistry is of an individual. If he finds an imbalance, then he will proceed to make the proper changes to bring the body back into balance, such as the acid/alkaline of the small intestine or of the stomach or colon. If the body is toxic and this toxicity is making the imbalance, then steps are taken to detoxify the person. If a person is deficient in particular vitamins or minerals, then those are supplemented. Periodic testing is then done to see if the assigned program is working for that individual. Mind and spirit therapy may also be a part of the patient's program.

3. How and why is a person detoxified?

Dr. Harold Manner once stated that most cancer patients have an average bowel movement of once every nine days and that a man one time came to him from one of the well-known institutes where he had surgery for his cancer. Dr. Manner asked him if they ever asked him about his bowel movements and he said no, all they did was cut on his tumor. Most cancer patients are very poisoned, very toxic and the first thing that they do in these clinics is to clean them out—maybe with laxatives, colonics, or coffee enemas. A three-day fast may be recommended, with juices. Carrot juice is used quite often, also apple and green juices. Some herbal medication may be given for the person's parasites. In some clinics they may treat the person for VD, TB and allergies. The patient may be sent to the dentist. The silver fillings may be replaced with oyster shell or some other, less toxic substance. They may be counseled for emotional detoxification. They may be counseled concerning their external environment. Whether they are using hair dyes, a deodorant that has aluminum in it, type of clothing they are using and substances in their house. Aluminum cookware would be discarded. Air purifiers and water purifiers may be recommended. Tinted eye glasses would be discarded and/or replaced with full spectrum. All this is done to help the body's immune system to function at its highest possible level.

4. How many clinics are there in Tijuana that treat cancer in this way?

There may be many clinics that treat cancer metabolically in Tijuana. The ones mentioned in this book are the ones that I am aware of. I am constantly researching clinics and it would not surprise me if Tijuana becomes the metabolic clinics capital of the world, if it isn't already.

5. Do all the clinics have real medical doctors?

Yes. There are staff and/or on-call doctors at all clinics.

6. What are the differences between these clinics?

Some of the clinics may use herbal formulas, some may use Laetrile, chelation therapy, ozone, immunology. Some use coffee enemas, some use a combination of some of these things. Most of them have a very special diet, a cleansing diet. American Biologics, Baja Hospital, Genesis West, Hospital Santa Monica, Manner and

Rosarita Beach are in-patient clinics. Bio-Medical and St. Jude's are out-patient clinics.

7. How are these clinics alike?

Most of them use a program for metabolic therapy, a detoxification program, a change of diet, a change of way of life. Most of the clinics recommend freshly grown, organically grown fruits and vegetables. All programs concentrate on cleansing the body and building the immune system.

8. Can these therapies be used along with orthodox treatment?

Yes, under the supervision of a physician.

9. Do any of these clinics use surgery, radiation and/or chemotherapy?

Yes. Four of them do, American Biologics, Hospital Ernest Contreras, and Manner Clinics.

10. Can these therapies be used with each other?

Yes, most of the time under the supervision of a physician.

11. Does one clinic have better success than the other?

This is really a difficult question to answer since these therapies must be continued at home and depend upon the individual's discipline and because many people combine these therapies. It is almost impossible, at this time, to be able to pick one clinic as being more successful, overall, than the rest. This is better described in the book, Cancer Control Society's Statistical Registry, 1984.

12. Does one clinic do better with certain types of cancer than another?

Certain clinics do claim to have success with certain types of cancer. Contreras Clinic seems to be quite successful with prostate cancer. Gerson and Manner Clinics seem to do quite well with brain tumors.

13. Do these doctors of the clinics meet with one another to discuss treatments and/or patients' recovery?

Unfortunately, at this time in 1995, the doctors are not having regular meetings with each other. They meet on occasion or maybe at a convention. They are beginning to go on the bus tour with us when we go on our Tijuana Clinics Tour and are beginning to observe how the other guy is doing, which is really going to be beneficial to all of us in the future.

14. Are there other clinics around the world that use metabolic therapy?

Yes. There are many.

15. Where can a person get a list of these clinics?

You can get a book written by John Fink, President of International Cancer Victors and Friends in Santa Barbara: P.O. Box 30493, Santa Barbara, CA 93105, (805) 969-9157.

16. What is a regular day of treatment in Mexico like?

Depending upon which clinic, of course, the treatment may vary. But in general it is very much like going to the doctor here in the United States. You may be given a blood test, a urine test and, in addition, you may be given a test that is not generally used here in the United States, such as a hair analysis. Patients are asked to bring with them any recent test results they may have to avoid retesting. X-raying a cancer patient over and over again may add to their chances of making things worse for themselves, so if the patient can bring their X-rays with them, this is helpful.

17. What is the average length of stay at the various clinics?

Most of the clinics want you to stay at the clinics or nearby to the clinics for three weeks. It is thought that during this time the body can be, generally, detoxified. A program for that patient can pretty well be established. The physicians can tell if this program is working, and if not can make any changes that need to be made, and the patients can learn what to do and what not to do for themselves when they return home. The patient is usually advised to seek out a metabolic physician near to where they live and asked to return to the Tijuana clinic, usually in two or three months, depending upon the severity of the case. The Hoxsey Clinic is the only one-day treatment. People can come without an appointment any day during the week as long as they arrive before 9:00 a.m. They are given blood and urine tests, a very thorough physical examination and by that night they have their medications, their vitamins and herbal formulas. They can be given a large enough supply of these for up to six months.

18. What is the average length of treatment?

One year to life. At the American Metabolic Clinic, they believe that the body can be detoxified and directed towards recovery in one year. CHIPSA Hospital, using the Gerson therapy, believes that the liver and pancreas must be rebuilt and that this takes a year and a half. It is thought that cancer, in general, is a very slow and progressive disease that has taken years to really establish itself in the body before it finally shows up as a tumor. Therefore, it is also thought that the length of treatment, to be non-toxic, is going to take time to reverse that situation and that there is, in most cases, time to do this. (If a tumor is pressing on a vital organ or obstructing an airway and detoxification cannot reduce that tumor fast enough, then radiation or surgery may be used—the radiation in small doses.) When it is said that it is a lifetime treatment, most of the clinics try to re-educate their patients to learn how to live in a different lifestyle to prevent their getting cancer again. So this becomes a lifetime effort.

19. How are the patients in the clinics followed up?

Hospital Ernesto Contreros, the Gerson Clinic and the Manner Clinics have their own methods of follow-up, but in general the clinics are not staffed for such procedures. In the United States cancer is the only disease that is followed, with the exception of a few other special diseases that are being researched. This cancer follow-up is usually done with a Tumor Registry. These registries can run hundreds of thousands of dollars.

20. Do these clinics only treat cancer?

No. Some of the clinics specialize in M.S. and arthritis, like the Manner Clinic. Some of the clinics treat all diseases. Dr. Contreras has a clinic and a hospital which is used also by the people in Mexico; it is not just people from America going there. They are fully staffed with doctors and nurses and this is the way it is with many of the clinics. They are seeing patients all of the time; they are not just cancer patients. A person may just go in for a physical examination. The physicians that work in these clinics are licensed physicians and licensed nurses treating different diseases.

21. Do any of these clinics treat AIDS?

Yes, American Biologics. Most of the other clinics do not have separate in-patient facilities for treating AIDS. Arrangements may be made with Bio-Medica, Contreres and the Manner Clinic for one day counseling and nutritional supplements.

22. Author's comment about a new kind of disease.

I want to add one thing to these questions and answers that I feel is urgent—and that is concerning all of the drug addiction here in the United States. I have always felt that the Gerson Therapy could be used for this because people who have gone there for their cancer have gotten off their morphine in about three or four days. There was a boy, who is now 30 years old, that apparently thought the same thing about the Gerson Therapy. At the age of 10 he was smoking cigarettes, at the age of 14 he was an alcoholic, at 18 using cocaine, at 21 heroin. Charlotte Gerson said, "I don't know how he got hold of this therapy, but he did. And now he says that he is no longer addicted to any of these drugs and, what is more, he said that he has no more cravings. His body is balanced nutritionally and he is not hungry for anything nor craving anything. Once that body has been balanced and is fed with the proper food, it has energy, it does not need any additional stimulants or relaxants." I would highly suggest that if you do have anyone in your family or know of someone that has alcohol or drug addiction, that you encourage them to contact the Gerson Clinic for more information. The Gerson Clinic also treats Alzheimer's Disease successfully. It may be that any of these clinics would have some success in these areas because all of them are concerned with cleansing the body. I mentioned the Gerson Therapy because of successful documented case histories.

23. Some people ask me how long I've been involved with alternative medicine.

I've been interviewing patients and alternative physicians for over 23 years.

24. And they wanted to know how I first got involved with Cancer Control.

I have five friends, one of them a physician, who had cancer. And it seemed to me that there were people all around me getting cancer and they were dying and they were using orthodox therapy. But I did have one friend who was using Kribiozen, a non-toxic substance (appearing not be damaging to the host or body), and she was surviving. I became quite interested, and when a physician friend of mine got cancer I began to search for alternatives. This physician friend also had refused orthodox therapy and a search for the alternatives seemed the only thing to do.

I did not know enough about alternatives to be of help to this friend and after his death I became more involved, wanting to know what would work, what could work, what might work. I knew that orthodox therapies were limited and I began to study about them and I began to help out at the Cancer Control Society. I would clip newspaper clippings and I would help out by making the biographies for the conventions and I began to see truth. I would see people the next year at the convention who had cancer, and they were still living, they were still walking around and I knew that there was something to this. We began to have tours to the Tijuana clinics and I would play hostess for the tours. Then I felt the tour needed, maybe, to have a little booklet of some kind to describe where we were going and I wrote the "Tijuana Clinics" and it turned out to be, with each update, a little larger, and it became a book. Then I wrote two other books, one about Wheatgrass Therapy and the other one, the *Alternative Cancer Therapy Study* 1984, on 111 patients using metabolic therapy. Anyone interested in getting a copy of any of the books can send for them from Alternative Cancer Therapies, 1803 Pacific Coast Highway, #5, Hermosa Beach, CA 90254.

25. People ask me how did I know how to do the statistics for the Cancer Control Society?

For three years I attended college at Cypress College, going for an accredited record technician degree. That is a degree in medical records. The statistics that I did are as near to how they would have been done had they been done here in the United States, considering the circumstances that I had to work with.

26. I've been asked if I'm going to continue to run this registry on a regular basis with a yearly report?

At present (1987) the Cancer Control Society doesn't have enough funding to carry on the Registry. With the money that they did receive for this purpose in 1985, which was about $700, I wrote to Nancy Reagan asking for her help in finding a grant for $25,000. Along with this letter I sent a copy of the Tijuana Clinics book and a copy of the Statistical Registry Report and a tape. A copy of the letter to Nancy was sent to all of the governors' wives (50 states) along with the two books and a tape. I received back from the White House a form letter thanking me for being concerned for the President's health. From the governors' wives, I received nothing. I then sent to 12 other sources for a grant, sources like the Ford Foundation and the Rockefeller Foundation. Three sent back negative replies. The other remaining, I have heard nothing from them. This was two years ago. It was stated in a German newspaper that our President, Ronald Reagan, had consulted with one of our metabolic physicians who is on the Cancer Control Society's Green Sheet, Dr. Hans Nieper, from Hanover, Germany. He is a doctor known for using metabolic therapy and even using Laetrile. And of course we want to try and get all of this here in the United States for the rest of us.

27. How do I see metabolic therapy being used here in the United States in the future?

Vitamins became popular during the First World War when they were sent to our boys overseas as a supplement for K-rations. This supplement was sent to make up for what wasn't in the cans. Now there are a lot of things that are not in our foods that we need, and there are a lot of things in our foods that we don't need. I believe that metabolic therapy is the only answer to this major problem. With the onset of many diseases and some new diseases—and you will see many more because of the way the food is bring processed—the way that they are radiating foods just to kill the bugs in it, the energy is being taken out of our foods. With the soils being depleted and all those additives, artificial flavorings and colorings and the salt, we are going to have to look more to metabolic therapy and more to prevention. I think that this just has to come about, just for our survival.

28. Do I see metabolic therapy as a financial benefit or financial threat to the United States?

I think in view of the DRG's (the Diagnostic Related Groups), and our Medi-Cal patients (our older patients) I would think that the United States would be very anxious to start incorporating metabolic therapy into their treatments and to keep our people well so that we won't have to be in debt. A lot of that Medi-Cal is going for medical services. Much of that funding, a lot of that money, is for that. Of course there is a lot of money being made off the chemotherapy and the radiation treatments—the cancer patients pay maybe $250,000 to be treated here. I think the cost and the insurance premiums are going to be so enormous in the future that no one is going to be able to afford it if it keeps on going up at the rate it is going. Even Medi-Cal has to be supplemented. We have to turn to metabolic therapy and to prevention. I think that when we do finally turn to prevention and metabolic therapy, our people are going to be working longer in their jobs; they are going to be happier, healthier. They are going to be more productive for a longer period of time; they are going to be able to earn more money longer. It's going to be a greater benefit to everyone.

29. What are the difficulties of metabolic therapy?

Most of our medical treatment here in the United States is that you can go to your doctor and he will examine you, give an injection, a prescription. Say that you get a cold: You feel sick, you go to the doctor, you get a shot, you go home, you get your pills. It is really hard for people to understand that a long time ago, when you got sick you went home, you rested, you might have had soup, and it took you a little bit longer to get over just a simple cold. But you could do it. And the same way it is with cancer, any disease; the rest is needed. What is really needed here in the United States is Cancer Sanitariums. We don't have anything like that; we want to go in and get the tumor cut off and come back home with our prescription and everything will be okay. It is just not realistic. Oh, we've been doing it, but it is not working. It's obviously not working. What is needed is a long-term type of sanitarium, a place for people to rest, a place for them to detoxify, to re-evaluate their lives and their lifestyles. To start to really look at what they are putting into their bodies, putting on their bodies, their environment. To make these changes mentally as well as physically during this time of mending the body. And of course we don't have insurance to pay for such a thing as of this date. We only have hospitalization which is very, very expensive. So most people who choose the metabolic therapy go home and hopefully they have someone to help them and they have a lot of discipline and they are able to follow a program for a year to a year-and-a-half and they can stay well. Many times the reason a metabolic therapy doesn't work is because the patient is unable to follow the program. It is too much for them to change so completely and so quickly and they don't have help.

30. What is wrong with alternative or metabolic therapy?

Alternative Medicine is an art and a science and because we are all different, can hardly be a mathematical equation, but still there is expected of most medicine to present some type of study, especially in regard to cancer statistics. Because of the numerous and combined and international therapies, no substantial tumor registry studies have been effectively implemented for Alternative Therapies in Mexico. Therefore, the patient seeking therapy in Mexico may have to do their own investigations, seek out counseling in regard to which clinic would be the wisest for them to go to.

31. What is the most asked question of someone seeking metabolic therapy?

"How do I know what thing to use and how do I know which one of these therapies is going to work and if it's going to work for me? Why are these therapies all different? Why aren't they the same? How do I know if I spend this money it won't be wasted? How do I know?" I tell patients: You know, you have to see what you're doing now. If you're not doing anything at all for yourself now, then you'll never know. And you have to study these different therapies and hopefully you know yourself well enough to know which one of these therapies you're going to be able to follow. Are you going to be able to drink carrot juice several times a day? Are you going to be able to not eat meat for a while? Are you going to be able to drink this herbal formula? Which therapy are you going to be able to handle mentally, emotionally? Do you have help? Do you have someone to help you with these therapies? I always tells people: You know you aren't doing anything at all right now. Pick a therapy, pick something and do something for yourself. If you improve the quality of your life just one little bit—just something for the next week, for the next day—then you have improved the quality of your life, you have done something to feel a little bit better. For that one day you have felt just a little bit better. So you haven't lost anything. You really haven't lost anything in just trying to go that one day, that one week. Get tested all the time. Know what's happening to your body. You don't want to be like at the races and pick a horse: You don't know whether it's going to come in or not, of course, but do something. Pick a therapy, start it, be tested all the time. If you find it's working according to the test, stay with that therapy. If you find that you need something else, look for something else. Incorporate something else, but all the time keep striving to do something.

32. Are there tests that a person can take to see if they have cancer?

Yes. There are some tests that can tell if you have the potential of getting cancer eight years ahead of the actual symptom, a tumor. The Neuhoeffer Test is given at the Hoxsey Clinic. The Navarro Test is a test you can mail to the Philippines for. The Neuhoeffer Test is $50 and the Navarro Test is $20. These tests are available. For more about tests and where to send for them, turn to PART VII.

33. Are these tests only given to people who think or know that they have cancer?

No. Many people take these tests on a regular basis because they don't want to get cancer. They are considered cancer markers. They are warnings.

34. What is the treatment for a test that shows positive?

The same as for the symptom of cancer, but usually to a lesser degree.

35. Are these tests used in the United States?

Yes. Some precancer tests are available. What isn't available can be sent for.

36. How can a person find out more about these tests and a doctor to give them?

(see PART IX)

37. Do you have any suggestions for a person who has found out that they have cancer?

Yes. First of all, find yourself a metabolic physician near to where you live, one that will work with you and your regular doctor. Take a tour to the Tijuana clinics. Read a lot about cancer and nutrition. Go to one of their conventions. Go to the National Health Federation Conventions. Talk to other patients who have used metabolic therapy for their cancer or their disease. Most of all, read, read, read all you can about cancer and nutrition.

38. What would you suggest to a person who doesn't have cancer and doesn't want to get it?

It is the same thing as if you have cancer. You should find a metabolic and nutritional doctor and be tested and read as many books as you can.

39. If a person has cancer, how can they decide which clinic in Tijuana to go to?

This is probably the most important decision that patients make regarding their metabolic care. I feel that any of these therapies may benefit a patient to a degree, but what is more important is to determine if a certain clinic has had good results with the particular type of cancer the patient has, and to determine the ability of the patient to follow a clinic's particular prescribed therapy. It is important that the patient has a hand in making the decision and a positive attitude and willingness to follow the therapy. Help in making these decisions can be obtained from Alternative Cancer Therapies, 1803 Pacific Coast Highway, Hermosa Beach, CA 90254, in talking with other patients, in researching through the available literature and by touring the clinics. If a tour is not available at the time, you may want to check into a motel in San Yisdro on this side of the border and make daily investigations of the clinics. If you stay at the International Motor Inn and R.V. Park at 190 E. Calle Primera (619) 428-4489 or at Days Inn, 225 Bay Blvd. (619) 425-8200, they will take you across the border the following day to the clinic that you wish to visit and bring you back later in the day. This is a service provided by the motels for patients staying in their facilities. They may go back and forth several times a day to the out-patient and in-patient clinics in Tijuana.

40. If a person has decided on a clinic in Tijuana, how can they get there?

If a patient already knows which therapy they are going to be taking and which clinic they are going to be going to, arrangements can sometimes be made with the clinic to be picked up at the border, the airport, or the bus station. For a patient who is going to a clinic that is an out-patient clinic, they may decide upon staying at the International Motor Inn, Days Inn or another nearby motel on this side of the border or in Tijuana.

41. How much does it cost to stay at these clinics?

To stay at American Biologics the cost is about $4,000 a week. At Bio-Medical the cost is $3,500 for term of illness (out-patient). Genesis West is $3,600 for a week. Hospital Santa Monica is about $2,500. Manner Clinic is about $3,000 for the week. Prices are subject to change. Dental care at the Morales Clinic is substantially lower than in the United States.

42. Will American medical insurance pay for these therapies?

Yes, depending upon which insurance company and whether it covers out of the United States. In general, most tests are covered. Some supplemental insurances for Medi-Cal are being honored. Visa and MasterCard are accepted at some of the clinics. To find out more about whether your particular insurance will pay for treatment at the clinics in Mexico please call or write to the following insurance coordinators: North American Insurance Coordinators, 5847 San Felipe Road, # 4200, Houston TX, 77057-3011, 7139530906. International Health Care Research, 895 Palomar Street, #A, Chula Vista, CA 91911, 619-575-7684. (See also PART VII)

What about Steve McQueen and Chad Green?

I have often heard, "Steve McQueen and Chad Green went to Mexico for treatment, and look what happened to them." Some people won't even hear about metabolic therapy, let alone consider it, because of these two people, which is too bad. The Chad Green and Steve McQueen stories are really success stories. Both Chad and Steve, according to orthodox medicine, were suffering from terminal illnesses. At best, the least that could have really been expected was to improve the quality of their lives, and metabolic therapy did that for them. Under their own individual circumstances, to have expected a cure for either one of them would have been a miracle according to modern medicine.

In America we have a tendency to want to speed things up and metabolic therapy is a slow process. Steve McQueen, although improving on metabolic therapy, decided to go to another place in Mexico to have a five-pound tumor removed from his stomach. He died from a heart attack as a result of the surgery.

Chad Green was lonely for his home town, his grandparents and his dog. If you have ever read about the psychological correlation between leukemia and loss of love objects, you can see that Chad lost several love objects. We will never know whether or not he could have been able to live longer had he been able to stay here in America and have metabolic therapy. It is almost certain that it would have been a lot less stressful on him.

PART VI

"And when one of you falls down he calls for those behind him, a caution against the stumbling stone. Ay, and he falls for them ahead of him who though faster and surer of foot, yet removed not the stumbling stone."
—Kahlil Gibran

Travel Information

TIJUANA CLINICS BUS TOURS

For information regarding available bus tours call the National Health Federation (818) 357-2181.

TRAVELING BY CAR

There are three important things to remember when traveling by car to Mexico: 1) Obtain car insurance preferably before or right after you enter Mexico. 2) Have proper identification with you for returning to the states. 3) Have legal papers and/or prescriptions for any medication being brought back into the United States.

CAR INSURANCE

The Mexican government does not recognize any foreign insurance. If you have an accident in Mexico, it is considered a felony. You must prove immediately financial responsibility for an accident. This can only be done by paying cash or by producing an approved Mexican insurance policy. You and your automobile could be impounded if you are not covered. This should not be discouraging. It is just a law of their country.

PROPER IDENTIFICATION

This should be in the form of a driver's license or a birth certificate. A driver's license is usually sufficient.

LEGAL PAPERS FOR MEDICATIONS

Legal forms for importing medication into the United States usually can be obtained from the clinic of the prescription. In most cases the prescription from the prescribing physician is sufficient.

OTHER INFORMATION

If you are traveling further south than Tijuana on the Ensenada Toll Road, you will be asked to pay a toll charge every so many miles. There are three of these toll stations to Ensenada. Each station will charge a little more than the previous one.

AMERICAN CONSULATE

In Tijuana 6-1001-05 or 6303-06 from 8:00 a.m. to noon and from 1:00 p.m. until 5:00 p.m. After-hours hotline is 8-2201 or 81-74-00. Agent 5124.

MEDICAL TRAVEL ASSISTANCE

4925 University Drive, #70, Huntsville, Alabama. (800) 828-8049.

WHERE TO STAY — International Motor Inn

International Motor Inn and RV Park (Motel 8) 190 E. Calle Primera San Ysidro, CA 92073 (619) 428-4489—a place with a unique service.

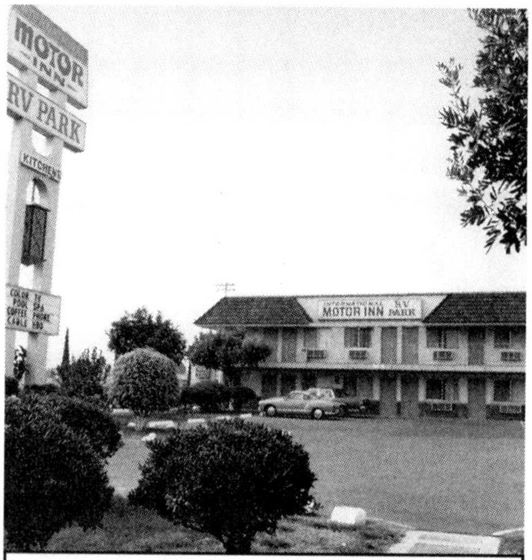

International Motor Inn and RV Park

For years patients have been staying at the International Motor Inn and RV Park (Motel 8). What makes this motel different from all the rest? There are two reasons:

1) When patients arrive in San Ysidro, they can call the International Motor Inn and the motel's manager, will have someone pick them up near the Greyhound Station and bring them back to the Motor Inn.

2) For more than fifteen years the Inn has employed drivers for the sole purpose of transporting patients across the border to the various clinics. The drivers work all day, crossing the border five to seven times a day, six days a week.

Patients usually arrive the day before their appointments at the clinics. The following morning at 7:00 a.m. they are taken by bus across the border to the clinic of their choice. After their visit to the clinic, they are picked up and returned to the Motor Inn. This service is completely free to the Motor Inn's patrons.

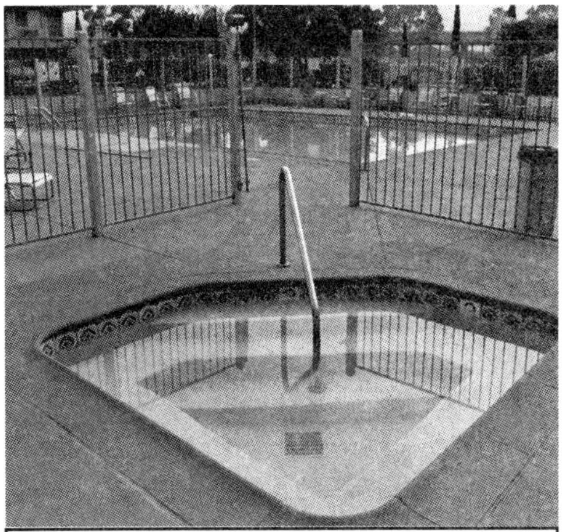

Pool Area

The first driver, Raul Coria, says that when he started out he drove a station wagon, but there were too many people and now they have several small buses.

Raul is a caring person and enjoys his work. He is very smart because he always says, "God bless all of you." And they always say, "God bless you too, Raul."

In addition to the International Motor Inn is another motel offering shuttle service to the Tijuana clinics. Their name and address: Days Inn, 225 Bay Blvd., Chula Vista, CA 91910, (619) 425-8200 and (800) 453-3297.

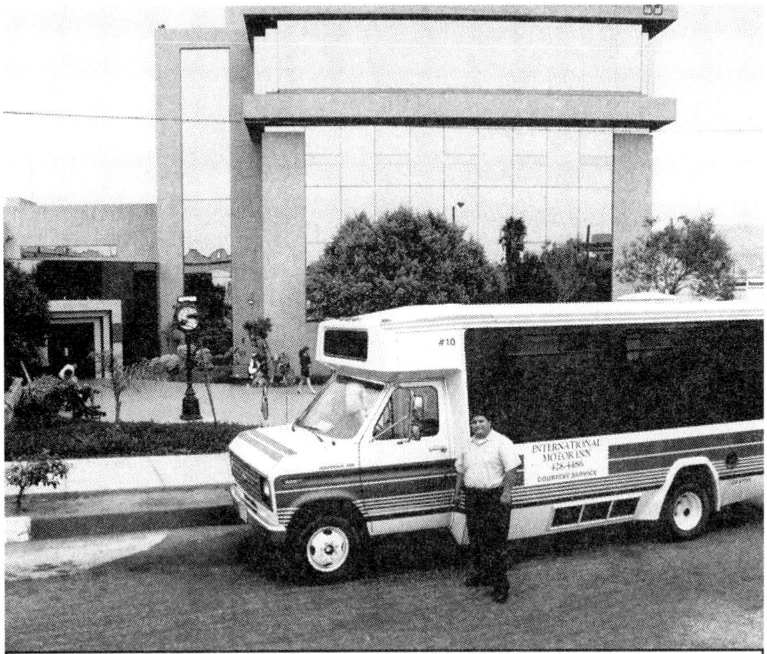

International Motor Inn Transport Bus

PART VII

"The annual Cancer Control Society Convention is very important to everybody—it keeps us informed on how to prevent or treat cancer. Thank you for this opportunity."
—Mary I. Nunez, R.N.

Health Societies

International Cancer Victors and Friends

How great it is. But, how did it all get started? Cecile Hoffman, a cancer patient, felt that she had made the discovery that Laetrile could keep her cancer under control and that this knowledge should be known and available to everyone. In 1963 she opened a small information center in San Diego, California. This information center was known as the International Association of Cancer Victims and Friends.

IACVF Active Chapter List

CALIFORNIA

- Santa Barbara Chapter, John Fink, Pres.,
  P.O. Box 30493, Santa Barbara, CA 93105
  805-969-9157
- Northern California Chapter, Grace Moore, R.N., Pres.
  5336 Harwood Rd., San Jose, CA 93105
  408-269-7466
- Montery Bay Chapter, Marene Mayer, Pres
  2578C El Camino Real N., Salinas, CA 93907
  408-663-5600
- West Los Angeles Chapter, Merri Cinquina
  7740 W. Manchester Blvd., #110, Playa del Rey, CA 90293
  213-306-0748

FLORIDA	▪ Palm Beach Chapter, Isolde Boutwell, Pres. P.O. Box 15102, West Palm Beach, FL 33416 407-798-4536, 407-969-2810
	▪ Central Florida Chapter, Harry Koontz, Pres. 5774 Chipola Circle, Orlando FL 32809 407-859-1931
	▪ Broward County Chapter, Pat Brett, Pres. P.O. Box 175, Fort Lauderdale, FL 33302 305-733-9121, 305-946-2770
	▪ Dade County Chapter, Rita Rauchwerger, Pres. P.O. Box 651285, Miami, FL 33165 305-271-2865
GEORGIA	▪ Atlanta Chapter, Hannah Feinreich, Pres. 1066 Ralph Road, Atlanta, GA 30324 404-634-4101, 404-426-4399
ILLINOIS	▪ Chicago Chapter, Terrie W. Wosnicki, Pres. 5508 W. 19th Street, 1-W, Cicero, IL 60650 708-780-6188
	▪ Niles Chapter, Dan Caddell, Pres. P.O. Box 48096, Niles, IL 60648 708-692-2596
NEVADA	▪ Las Vegas Chapter, Aimee Alterwitz, Pres. 5235 Chiefton Street N., Las Vegas, NV 89129 702-795-4868
NEW JERSEY	▪ New Jersey Chapter, Herb Horky, Pres. 12 Van Ethel Drive, Matawan, NJ, 07747 201-583-1274
NEW YORK	▪ Long Island Chapter, Maxine Hubbs Levine, Pres. 481 Division Ave., Hicksville, NY 11801 516-796-3964
TEXAS	▪ Amarillo Chapter, Bryan Denson, Pres. 3600 Amherst, Amarillo, TX 79109 806-355-7782
	▪ El Paso Chapter, Faye LaRue, Pres. P.O. Box 3294, El Paso, TX 79923 915-755-0724
WASHINGTON	▪ Seattle Chapter, Matthew Kulawiee, Pres. 3706 231st. Street, S.E., Bothell,WA, 98011 206-481-4351
CANADA	▪ Victoria Chapter, Bruce Reid, Pres. P.O. Box 6502 Depot 1, Victoria, B.V. V8P 5M4 478-8156
AUSTRALIA	▪ Melbourne Chapter, Robin Bailey, Pres. 250 Union Road, Surrey ills, Vic. 3127 03-836-8764

Other Organizations

- ACT-UP/NEW YORK, 496A Hudson Street, N.Y., N.Y. 10014 (212) 989-1114 Eastern time. Send $8.00 for a 100-page booklet on Alternatives and Holistic AIDS Treatment Options. Also includes information on the politics of holistic health care, alternative theories about the causes of AIDS (not all believe it is the HIV virus) and local resources.
- CAN HELP (206) 437-2291 Pacific time. A service that helps people with cancer find the best treatments, both within and outside mainstream medicine. For $400, you will receive a customized computer search of the worldwide medical literature by journalist Patrick M. McGrady, Jr. who is available by phone to discuss the report.
- CANCER CHRONICLES, 161 West 61st Street, Suite 5B, N.Y., N.Y. 10023. Send $12 for a yearly subscription to this quarterly newsletter to keep up on Emprise, the OTA report, and other issues raised at this conference.
- THE CANCER INDUSTRY: Unravelling the Politics by Ralph Moss (New York: Paragon House 1989). A source for anyone interested in knowing how and why several promising alternative cancer therapies were discredited before full scientific evaluation. Available at bookstores or order directly by calling (800) PARAGON.
- CANCER SURVIVORS NEWSLETTER, P.O. Box 1221, Chula Vista, CA 91910.
- COMMUNITY RESEARCH INITIATIVE (212) 481-1050 Eastern time. Call to learn which AIDS drugs are being researched and how to take part. Will refer you to similar community-based projects in other cities.
- FANE, 7850 White Lane #E 341, Bakersfield, CA 93309 (805) 588-2397.
- HEAL (Health Education AIDS Liaison), 16 East 16th Street, N.Y., N.Y. 10003 (212) 674-HOPE Eastern time. Send $7 for a 100-page packet of reprints of articles on alternative approaches to strengthening the immune system. Send $10 for a one-year subscription to a quarterly newsletter about holistic treatments. HEAL refers to practitioners on both coasts, sponsors weekly support group meetings, and provides help in organizing a local chapter.
- HEALTH FACTS(r) ISSN 0738-811X is published twelve times a year by the Center for Medical Consumers, Inc., a non-profit organization. Arthur Aaron Levin MPH, Director. Offices are 237 Thompson Street, N.Y., N.Y., 10012 (212) 674-7105.

(c) The Center for Medical Consumers 1990. Special written permission is required to reproduce, in any manner, in whole or in part, the material contained within. Subscriptions are $18 for one year (U.S.A.). Back issues and bulk rates available upon request. Indexed by *Consumers Health and Nutrition Index.* Published quarterly by The Oryx Press.

- NATIONAL HEALTH FEDERATION (THE), (818) 357-2181 Pacific time. P.O. Box 688, Monrovia, CA 91016. Provides doctors and clinical lists for those seeking natural therapies, or an augmentation of their present therapy. The NHF keeps a library of articles on natural remedies and supplies books that are of help to those who are ready to take responsibility for their own health and the health of their families. NHF is strong in the belief that self education is paramount.
  Publications - Health Freedom News and Shedding Light on Legislation.

- PEOPLE AGAINST CANCER (515) 972-4444 Central time. Provides free phone consultation on a wide variety of alternative cancer therapies. PAC neither recommends practitioners nor treatments, rather it provides information upon which to make an informed decision. A position paper on the OTA report is planned. PEOPLE WITH CANCER, a subsidiary of PAC, lobbies for thc right to choose alternative cancer therapies and for insurance reimbursement.

- PROJECT CURE, a Washington, D.C. based group that works within the legislative process for freedom of choice. Call (800) 552-CURE, Eastern time for a free packet of articles on the politics of cancer and a free copy of the book, Repression and Reform in the Evaluation of Alternative Cancer Therapies by Robert G. Houston.

- THE VANGUARD SUPRESS, Inc. P.O. Box 10400, Glendale, CA 91209-3400 (818) 790-6383. Fax: (818) 790-9660.

PART VIII

"So eat always from the table of God: the fruits of the trees, the grain and the grasses of the field, the milk of the beasts, and the honey of the bees." —Jesus, Essene Gospel of Peace

What You Can Do

Immune Enhancer Check List

	yes	no
Whenever possible eat organically-grown fruits and vegetables.		
Eat raw foods whenever possible—25%, 50%, 75% of the time.		
Use filtered or order spring water.		
When cooking use only stainless steel or glass cookware.		
Use an air purifier and/or ionizer in home and/or office.		
Wear clothing made of natural fibers and fit comfortably.		
Use only hair and cosmetic products that contain non-allergic or non-toxic agents.		
Use deodorant that does not contain aluminum, hexachlorophene or other harmful ingredients.		
Use toothpaste that does not contain fluoride.		
Check household for toxic agents and remove.		
Have installed full-spectrum lighting indoors.		
Wear full-spectrum eye glasses.		
Go to bed early and get needed amount of sleep.		
Keep pets out of doors or have them placed in foster homes.		
Use natural herbicides on lawns or in gardens.		

Immune Enhancer Check List		
	yes	no
Consult with physician and metabolic physician on a regular basis.		
Have had a hair analysis test to check for toxic metals.		
Have had silver/mercury fillings removed and replaced with a lesser, non-toxic substance such as plastic or oyster shell.		
Have gone for emotional or spiritual counseling.		
Check house for radon levels. Electric company for EM's		
Health Education Check list		
I have joined health organization/s and/or receive a monthly health magazine.		
I attend health conventions at least twice a year.		
I read two health books a month.		
I have an alphabetical file (folders) on health.		
I visit health food stores once a month to see new books and products.		
I visit book stores and/or used book stores at least every two months.		
I regularly visit with someone who can teach me something new about health and I teach someone too.		
I have toured the Tijuana Clinics.		

Pharmaceuticals

- **Arterosclerosis Retinoparty**
  Biopharm
  Postfach 73057
  D-2000 Hamburg 73
  West Germany
- **Metabolic**
  American Biologics
  1180 Walnut Ave
  Chula Vista, CA 92011
  619-429-8200
  800-227-4473
- **Regeneration**
  C.P.W. Rahlstedt
  P.O. Box 73 or 27
  D-2000 Hamburg 73
  West Germany
  011-49-40-6770037
- **Dental Information**
  Health-Wise—Dental Wise
  639 Washington Street
  Columbus, IL 47201
  812-376-8525
- **Metabolic**
  Bio-Apotheke
  Inhaber Knaus
  Franentrasse 17
  8000 Munchen S
  West Germant
  089-225630
- **Vitamins, Minerals, Herbs, Books, Tapes, Pet Products**
  Whole Health Catalog
  P.O. Box 328
  Westville, OK 74965-0328
  800-562-7206

- **Black Walnut**
  American Biologics
  1180 Walnut Ave
  Chula Vista, CA 92011
  619-429-8200
  800-227-4473

- **Cloves**
  San Francisco Herb Co.
  Natural Food Company
  1010 46th Street and Adeline
  Emeryville, CA 94608
  800-277-2830

- **Enzymes**
  Enzyme Therapy
  P.O. Box 22310
  Green Bay, WI 54305
  800-783-2286

- **Herbs**
  Health Center for
  Better Living
  6189 Taylor Road
  Naples, FL 33942
  813-566-2611

- **Hydrogen Peroxide 35%**
  New Horizons Trust
  53166 State Route 681
  Reedville, OH45772
  800-755-6360

- **Iodine, Pure**
  Spectrum Chemical Company
  14422 South San Pedro Street
  Gardena CA 90248
  800-772-8786

- **Laetrile**
  Kem.S.A. Laboratories
  P.O.Box 1561
  Chula Vista, CA 92012
  011-53-66-806842

- **Magnesium Oxide**
  Bronson Pharmaceuticals
  4526 Rinetti Lane
  P.O. Box 628
  Lacanada, CA 91012
  800-722-3821

- **Metabolic**
  American Metabolics
  1180 Walnut Ave
  Chula Vista, CA 92011
  619-429-8200
  800-227-4473

- **Potassium Iodide, Pure**
  Spectrum Chemical Co.
  14422 South San Pedro St.
  Gardena CA 90248
  800-772-8786

- **Rodaquin**
  Ave. Madrid Y Oslo
  No. 42-B FRACC
  Costa Azul
  Palyas de Tijuana

- **Wormwood Combination**
  Koeger Herb Products
  805 Walnut Street
  Boulder, CA 80302
  800-225-8787
  303-443-0261

Insurance Companies

- Aetna Insurance Company, Utah, International, Inc., New Mexico
- Benefit Life Insurance Company, Wean United, Inc., Ohio
- Blue Cross & Blue Sheild of Southern California
- Blue Cross & Blue Shield of Pennsylvania
- Farm Bureau Health Program
- Cal Farm Life Insurance Company California
- The Guardian Life Insurance Company of America, West Virginia
- King County Medical Blue Shield, Washington
- Mail Handlers Benefit Plan, Maryland
- Lincoln National Life Insurance Company, California
- NN Investor Life Insurance Company, Inc., Texas

- Prudential Insurance Company of America, Florida
- Prudential Insurance Company of America, Minnesota
- Southwest Airlines Company, Health Benefits Trust, Texas
- Travelers
- Union Bankers Insurance Company, Dallas, Texas, Wisconsin

INSURANCE CO-ORDINATORS

- International Health Reasearch
  895 Palomar Street, #A
  Chula Vista CA 91911
  (619) 575-7684
- North American Health Insurance Co-ordinators
  5847 San Felipe Road, #4200
  Houston TX 77057-3011
  (713) 953-0906

Bibliography & Suggested Reading

Read! Read! Read!

CLINIC READING

- Contreras Therapy
  Too Young To Die, Rick Hill
- Genesis Therapy
  Andrew McNaughton Journal, Cancer Control Society
  Laetrile Diet Cook Book, Florence Joyce
- Gerson Therapy The Gerson Therapy—50 Case Histories, Dr. Max Gerson
  The Gerson Therapy Journal, Cancer Control Society
  Gerson Institute Journal "Healing", Vols 1 & 2
  Cancer Winner, Jackie Davison
- Hoxsey Therapy
  You Don't Have To Die, Harry Hoxsey
- Integrated Therapy
  International Protocols (IIMP) In Cancer Management, Bradford, Culbert Allen
- Manner Therapy
  The Death of Cancer, Dr. Harold Manner
  Manner Metabolic Therapy Journal, Cancer Control Society
  Manner Metabolic "C," Dr. Harold Manner
- Donsbach Therapy
  Any book by Dr. Kurt Donsbach.

OTHER SUGGESTED READING

- Learn more about alternative medicine! Read the following books! Most of them are available from: The

National Health Federation P.O. Box 688 Monrovia, CA 91016 (818) 357-2181.

- The Bodhi Tree Phoenix Bookstore 8585 Melrose Avenue West Hollywood, CA and Santa Monica, CA (310) 659-1733
- San Diego Controversial Book Store 3021 University Avenue San Diego, CA (619) 296-1560
- Libraries, Book Stores, Unusual and Rare Book Stores, and Health Food Stores
- Appleton, Nancy, Ph.D., Lick The Sugar Habit
- Asai, Kazuniko, Ph.D., Miracle Cure, Organic Germanium
- Bailey, H., Gerovital (GH3) Will It Keep/Young Longer
- Baker, E., Uncook Book
- Borderland Sciences Research Fdt., Koch Remedy/Cancer
- Brandt, Joanna, The Grape Cure
- Burk, Dean, Ph.D., Vit. B17, B15, B13, Brief Foods/Vits
- Carter, Albert, The Cancer Answer
- Chaitow, Leon, D.O., An End To Cancer
- Clark, Hulda, Cure For All Cancers, Cure For All Diseases, Cure For HIV & AIDS
- Cousins, Norman, Anatomy of An Illness
- Culbert, Mike, Freedom From Cancer
- Dadd, Debra Lynn, Non Toxic & Natural - Non-Toxic Home
- Dailin, Lynn, Ph.D., Cancer Causes & Natural Controls
- Diamond, John., M.D., Your Body Doesn't Lie
- Donsbach, K., Ph.D., Chelation Therapy - DMSO - Metabolic Cancer Therapies
- Duarte, Alex, O.D., Cataract Breakthrough
- Dufty, William, Sugar Blues
- Ericson, R., B.S., Cancer Treatment/What You Can Do
- Fink, John, Third Opinion (Alternative Therapy Directory)
- Fischer, William, How To Fight Cancer & Win

- Garten, Max, D.C., Diseases/Their Circumvention
- Gerson, Max, M.D., Cancer Therapy 50 Cases - Appendix to Older Edition
- Glassman, Judith, The Cancer Survivors
- Gofman, John, M.D., Ph.D., Radiation & Human Health
- Griffin, Edward, World Without Cancer
- Gutting, Robert, Chelation Therapy - Chromium - Glandulars - Hypoglycemia - Selenium
- Halstead, Bruce, M.D., Chelation Therapy - Amygdalin (Laetrile) Therapy - Metabolic Cancer Therapy - Scientific Basis of EDTA Chelation Therapy - Hyperbaric Oxygen Therapy
- Halstead, M.D. & Youngberg, DMSO Handbook
- Hamlyn, Edward, M.D., Healing Art of Homeopathy
- Haught, S.J., Cancer? Curable! The Gerson Therapy Health Research, Is Cancer Curable? (collection/reprints)
- Heinsohm, Douglas, Cancer, Metabolic Therapy, Laetrile
- Hill, Rick, Too Young To Die (breast cancer)
- Howell, Edward, Dr., Food Enzymes/Health & Longevity - Enzyme Nutrition
- Hoxsey, Harry, N.D., You Don't Have To Die
- Huggins, Hal, D.D.S., It's All In Your Head
- Hunter, Beatrice, Consumer Beware - Additive Book
- Huntington, Barbara, Cancer Patient's Survival Manual
- International Health Council, A Program for Prevention, Detection and Reversal of Pre-Cancerous Conditions
- Jensen, Bernard, D.C., Iridology Simplified - Doctor-Patient Handbook
- Julian, J., M.D., Chelation: Prevent Heart Attacks/Stroke
- Kelley, William, D.D.S., One Answer To Cancer
- Kime, Z., M.D., Sunlight Could Save Your Life
- Koch, Wm., M.D., Immunity & Oxidative Therapy - Survival Factor in Neoplastic & Viral Diseases - Neoplastic & Viral Parasitism

- Kuhnau, Wilfram, M.D., Live-Cell Therapy
- Laws, Pricilla, Ph.D., The X-ray Information Book
- Lee, Lita, Ph.D., Radiation Protection Manual
- Linde & Carrow, D., M.D., Directory of Holistic Medicine & Alternative Health Care Services in the U.S.
- Livingston, Virgina, M.D., Cancer: A New Breakthrough - Diet for Cancer - Patients Handbook - Microbiology of Cancer - Physician's Handbook - Conquest of Cancer
- Lynes, Barry, The Cancer Cure That Worked
- Lubecki, John, End of Cancer
- Manner, Harold, Ph.D., Manner Metabolic Therapy "C"-Metabolic Therapy "A" -Metabolic Therapy "B"
- Manning, Betsy Russell, How Safe Are Silver (mercury)/Nickel Fillings? - Candida, Silver (mercury) Fillings/Immune System
- Marx, Henry, GH3 in the Battle Against Old Age
- McBean, Eleanor, Vaccination Condemned
- McNaughton Fdt., Amygdalin-The Non-Toxic Analgesic - Laetrile-Nitrilosides/Prevention and Control of Cancer - Physician's Handbook/Vitamin B17 Therapy - Vit B15 Indications/Use/Efficacy/Internal Disease - Vit B15 (Pangamic Acid) Properties/Functions/Use
- Mindell, Earl, Vitamin Bible - Vitamin Bible For Your Kids
- Moscato, Tony, I Chose To Live
- Natenberg, Maurice, Cancer Blackout
- Newbold, H.L., M.D., Vitamin C Against Cancer
- Nieper, Hans, M.D., Dr. Nieper's Revolution
- Nolfi, Kristine, M.D., Raw Food Treatment Cancer/Other
- Oden, Clifford, Rev., Thank God I Had Cancer
- Ott, John, D.Sc., Hon., Color & Light - Ott Reprint - Light/Health CCJ - Light/Radiation/You
- Passwater, Richard, Ph.D., Cancer/Nutritional Therapies- Selenium/Food & Medicine
- Pauling, Ph.D., Cameron, M.D., Cancer & Vit C

- Price Weston, D.D.S., Nutrition & Physical Degeneration
- Prince, Pat, Contreras Clinic Laetrile Cookbook
- Rawls, Walter, Jr., Davis, Albert R., The Magnetic Effect
- Richardson, J., M.D. & Griffith, P., R.N., Laetrile Case Histories
- Roberts, Gordon, Cancer-How It May Be Wiped Out
- Rork, Mary Lee, Gerson Therapy Handbook
- Salaman, Maureen, Nutrition/The Cancer Answer
- Sartori, Hellfried, M.D., Cancer 1985
- Schauss, Alexander, Diet, Crime & Delinquency
- Schechter, Steven, N.D., Fighting Radiation With Foods
- Siegel, Bernie, M.D., Love, Medicine & Miracles
- Simmons, H., Psychogenic Biochemical Aspects/Cancer
- Simonton, Carl, M.D., Getting Well Again p/b
- Singer, Peter, & Mason, Jim, Animal Factories
- Stauth, Cameron, New Appproach To Cancer
- Stickle, Rbt., Cancer-One Man's Fight/Control Malignancy - A Rational Concept of Cancer
- Taylor, Renee, Hunza Health Secrets
- Van Strum, Carol, A Bitter Fog (Herbicides)
- Waerland, Ebba, Cancer, Disease of Civilization
- Wahi, Albert, M.D., Birth of A Science (Koch Therapy)
- Waldbott, George, M.D., Fluoridation Dilemma
- Walker, Morton, D.P.M., Chelation Therapy - How Not To Have a Heart Attack - Miracle Power/Chelation - Chelation Answer - Coping With Cancer - Garlic - Chelation
- Warburg, Otto, Ph.D., Causes & Prevention of Cancer
- Wead, Bill, Second Opinion (LaPacho & Cancer)
- Welch, Richard, M.D., New Hope for Cancer Victims
- Westover, Wynn, See The Patients Live

- Wigmore, Ann, Be Your Own Doctor - Why Suffer (Wheatgrass)
- Williams, Don, Dead by Now
- Winters, Jason, Killing Cancer & Perisel
- Wolper, Sally, Tijuana Clinics - Where & How To Go - Leukemia & Metabolic Therapy - AIDS INFO
- Wright, Jane, Diagnosis: Cancer (Burton Therapy)
- Yiamouyiannis, J., Ph.D., Fluoride-The Aging Factor
- Ziff, Sam, The Toxic Time Bomb (Ag/Hg Fillings)

ARTHRITIS BOOKS

- Adams, R. & Murray, F., Arthritis, New Hope For Sufferers
- Airola, Paavo, N.D., There is a Cure for Arthritis
- Alexander, Dale, Arthritis/Com. Sense No. 1 - No. 2
- Bingham, Robert, M.D., Fight Back Against Arthritis
- Campbell, G., D.O., Dr.'s Proven Home Cure/Arthritis
- Cobb, Lawrence, DMSO-The Myths & Facts
- Dong, Collin, M.D., Banks, Jane, Arthritic's Cookbook
- Fredericks, Carlton, Ph.D., Arthritis, Don't Learn To Live with It
- Ind. Cancer Research Fdt., Got a Horse? Get DMSO
- Jarvis, Bernard, D.C., Arthritis and Folk Medicine
- Jensen, Bernard, D.C., Overcoming Arthritis/Rheumatism
- Manner, Harold, Ph.D., Metabolic Therapy "A"
- McGrady, Pat., Sr., Persecuted Drug: Story of DMSO
- Wade, Carlson, Arthritis, Nutrition & Natural Therapy

MULTIPLE SCLEROSIS BOOKS

- East, Robert, Living Above It!
- Evers, P. & J., M.D.'s, 60 Recipes/MS/Metabolic Disease
- Graham, Judy, MS-A Self-Help
- Manner, Harold, Ph.D., Metabolic Therapy for MS
- Morrissette, Claire, Hope For Us (Neiper Therapy)
- Sartori, H.E., M.D., Multiple Sclerosis 1985
- Soll, Robert, M.D., MS Something Can Be Done -You Can Do It

ALTERNATIVE CANCER CONVENTION CASSETTES AND VIDEOS

- Convention Cassette Tapes and Videos List Available from TAPCO, P.O. Box 829, Lowell, AR 72745 (501) 770-0627.

PART IX

"One of the best ways to safeguard yourself from being deceived is always to form the habit of looking at things for yourself, listening to things for yourself, thinking for yourself, before you try and come to any judgement."—Malcolm X

TESTS

Some alternative cancer markers can indicate the probability of cancer eight years (Neunhoeffer) before the tumor appears. If a person's tests shows that there is a high probability of getting cancer, the person is given thymus shots and other immune enhancing therapies. They are then tested again and until the tests show that they are out of danger.

Hippocrates realized that diseases progressed in degrees. The Alternative Physician works to reverse disease in the same way, in degrees. These sophisticated tests are used to measure the progress of this reversal. Tests are given before, during and after treatment. This helps the physician to evaluate which therapy is most effective.

SOME TESTS CAN BE SENT FOR BY MAIL.

The following is a list of some of these tests:

- Neunhoeffer Test
  BioMedical Center P.O.Box 433654 San Ysidro, CA 92143 001-52-66-849011/849132 Eves.

- Manual D. Navarro, M.D.
  3553 Sining, Morningside Terr. Santa Mesa, Manilla 2806, Phillipines 61-26-92/61-42-68

- Hospital Ernesto Contreras
  P.O. Box 439045 San Ysidro, CA 800-326-1850
- Dietmar Schildwaechter, M. D.
  Sovereign Consultants International P.O. Box 16602 Dulles International Airport Washington, D.C. 20041 703-430-7789
- Healthexcel
  (Nutitional Evaluation) P.O..Box 495 Winthrop, WA 98862 509-996-213

FOR CLINICAL PRE-CANCER TESTING IN MEXICO:

- Hospital Ernesto Contreras
  P.O. Box 439045 San Ysidro, CA
  800-326-1850Contreras
- American Biologics 1180 Walnut Avenue Chula Vista, CA 92110-2622 (619) 429-8200
- Bio-Medical Center P.O.Box 433654 San Ysidro, CA 92143 001-52-66-849011/849132 Eves.

Directions

Thank you again for your
interest in this subject.
Good luck in your search
for perfect health.

DIRECTIONS TO THE CLINICS

- To Ernesto Contreras Hospital (Contreras Clinic) 1) Go around traffic loop 2) Continue on Carr Internacional or 3rd or 2nd street to Playas 3) When road starts to curve left, look for the Contreras Clinic and Pharmacy across from the bullring.
- To Hospital de CHIPSA (Gerson Clinic) 1) Go around traffic loop 2) Continue on Carr Internacional or 3rd and 2nd Street to Playas 3) When road starts to curve left, look for a pharmacy on the left and bullring on the right 4) Continue on road for about 1/2 mile and look for CHIPSA Hospital on the left.
- To Bio-Medical Center (Hoxsey Clinic) 1) Go around traffic loop 2) Drive three blocks to Ave Revolucion and turn left 3) When this turns left into Blvd. Agua Caliente, 4) Look for and turn right onto General Ferreira 5) Follow to Hoxsey—top of the hill on left.
- To Manner Clinic (Manner Therapy) 1) Go around traffic loop 2) Follow Carr Internacional or 3rd or 2nd Street 3) Look for the Mesa Posada Del Sol, 1/2 way up hill 4) Follow to Manner clinic near bridge and other freeway
- Driving Instructions to Hospital Santa Monica at Playa Santa Monica from the U.S./Mexican border crossing at Tijuana.

  Stay in the third lane from the right when crossing the border. Within 400 feet you will go through some arches. There should be a sign over the lane you are in which says "Ensenada Rosarito." Stay in this lane. Within ¼ mile, the lane turns to the left under an overhead sign which says "Ensenada Cuota" and makes a complete circle onto a one-way road. Within two miles the road climbs a steep hill and makes a left turn. On the other side of the hill, take the first road to the right onto a road heading west. Within a mile or so the road makes a left turn at the city of Playas de Tijuana (4.4 miles from the border). Within less than a ½ mile you will reach the toll booth (amount posted on the booth—less than $1 U.S.). After the toll booth the road divides and continues south along the ocean for the next 12.6 miles to the Rosarito exit. Just before Rosarito the road turns to the left and in a mile makes a sweeping turn to the right.

The exit is on your right within 300 feet and puts you on a two-way traffic street. Take the first road to your right (within 200 feet). It is paved. In less than a mile you will pass some oil tanks on your right. The road makes a right turn and within 500 feet becomes a dirt road. Continue for another mile until you reach a road on your left with a yellow, diamond-shaped road sign. Turn left on this road and go under an archway which says "Playa Santa Monica." Take the first road after the archway to your left (within 50 feet). Hospital Santa Monica is in front of you (two-story blue building). Park to the left alongside the building.

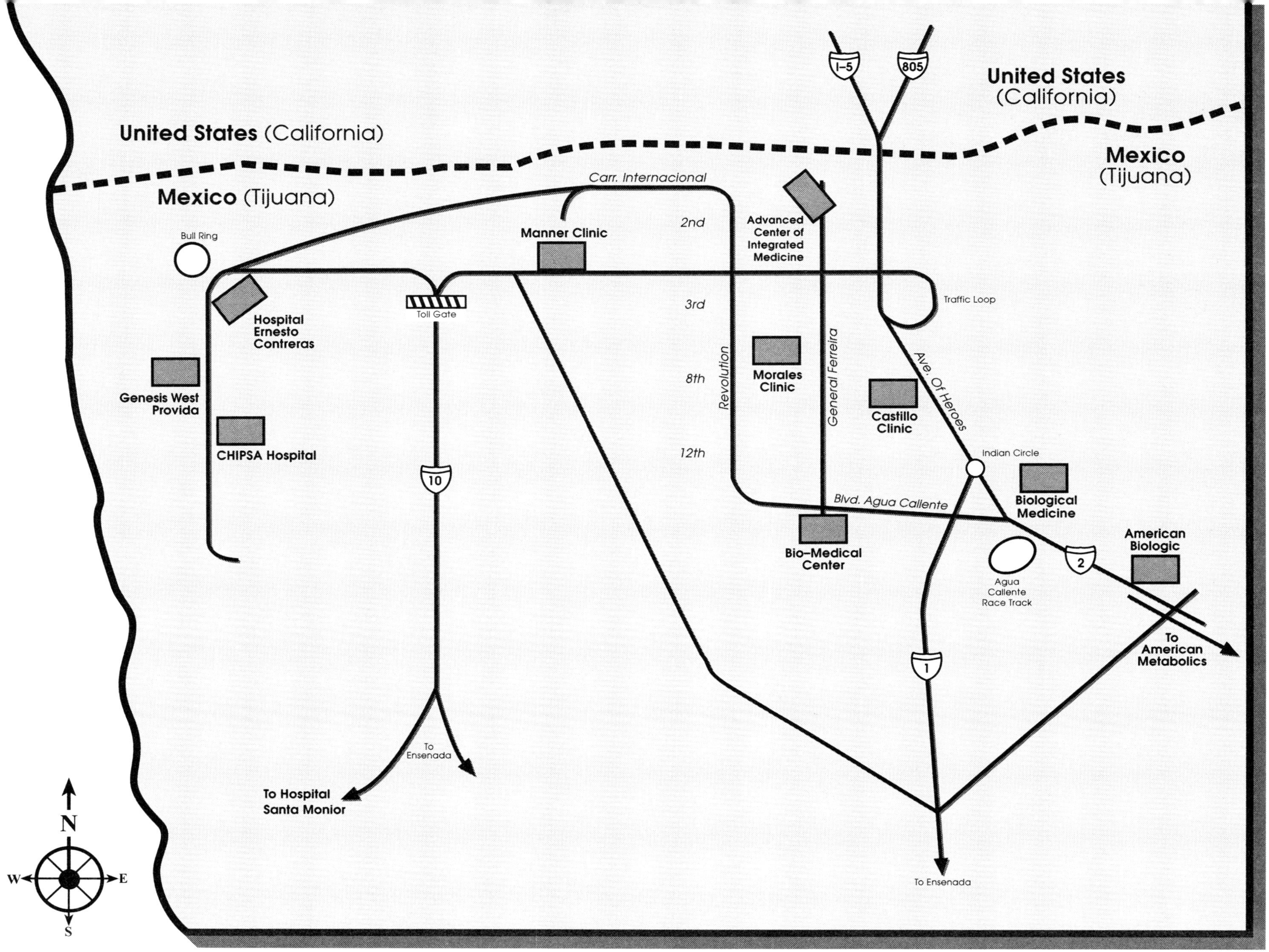
United States (California)
Mexico (Tijuana)
United States
(California)
Mexico
(Tijuana)
I-5
805
Carr. Internacional
Bull Ring
Manner Clinic
2nd
Advanced
Center of
Integrated
Medicine
Toll Gate
3rd
Traffic Loop
Hospital
Ernesto
Contreras
Genesis West
Provida
8th
Revolution
Morales
Clinic
General Ferreira
Castillo
Clinic
Ave. Of Heroes
CHIPSA Hospital
12th
Indian Circle
10
Biological
Medicine
Blvd. Agua Callente
Bio–Medical
Center
American
Biologic
2
Agua
Callente
Race Track
To
American
Metabolics
1
To
Ensenada
To Hospital
Santa Monior
To Ensenada
N
W
E
S

Notes